Pricing Life

Basic Bioethics
Glenn McGee and Arthur Caplan, editors

Pricing Life: Why It's Time for Health Care Rationing, Peter A. Ubel

Pricing Life
Why It's Time for Health Care Rationing

Peter A. Ubel, M.D.

A Bradford Book
The MIT Press
Cambridge, Massachusetts
London, England

First MIT Press paperback edition, 2001
© 2000 Massachusetts Institute of Technology

This book was set in Sabon by Wellington Graphics and was printed and bound in the United States of America.

Library of Congress Cataloging-in-Publication Data

Ubel, Peter A.
  Pricing life: Why it's time for health care rationing / Peter A. Ubel.
    p. cm.—(Basic bioethics series)
  "A Bradford book."
  Includes bibliographical references and index.
  ISBN 0-262-21016-9 (hc. : alk. paper), 0-262-71009-9 (pb)
    1. Health care rationing. 2. Medical care—Cost effectiveness. I. Title. II. Series.
  RA410.5.U533 1999
  362.1—dc21   99-20664
                                                                            CIP

Unless otherwise indicated, the cases presented in this book are hypothetical. Some are based on real cases or combinations of real cases, but names and medical facts have been changed to protect the identities of patients involved. The Coby Howard case from Oregon, however, is real, and the reports in this book are based on events that were well publicized in the media.

Much of the empirical research presented here was published previously. References are provided to indicate where specific studies appeared. In addition, several of the arguments developed in this book are extensions of published articles. Chapter 2 is an extension of an article from the *Archives of Internal Medicine*, "Rationing" health care: Not all definitions are created equal, 158:209–214, 1998. Chapter 4 is an extension of a paper from the *Kennedy Institute of Ethics Journal*, The challenge of measuring community values in ways appropriate for setting health care priorities (in press). Chapter 7 is based on an article in the *Annals of Internal Medicine*, Recognizing bedside rationing: Clear cases and tough calls, 126:74–80, 1997. Chapter 8 is based on an article from the *New England Journal of Medicine*, Rationing by any other name, 336:1668–1671, 1997.

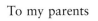

To my parents

Contents

Series Foreword

We are pleased to present the first volume in the series Basic Bioethics. The series presents innovative book-length manuscripts in bioethics to a broad audience and introduces seminal scholarly manuscripts, state-of-the-art reference works, and textbooks. Such broad areas as the philosophy of medicine, advancing genetics and biotechnology, end of life care, health and social policy, and the empirical study of biomedical life will be engaged.

Glenn McGee
Arthur Caplan

Basic Bioethics Series Editorial Board
Tod S. Chambers
Carl Elliot
Susan Dorr Goold
Mark Kuczewski
Herman Saatkamp

Acknowledgments

This book would not have happened without the help of many of my close colleagues and friends. Several parts of the book are extensions of work I published previously with other people. Susan Dorr Goold was extremely helpful in helping me think through the concepts I discuss in chapters 2, 3, and 7. Bob Arnold and I worked together in developing the ideas presented in chapters 6 and 9. David Asch and I worked together on the work described in chapter 8 and on much of the empirical research in chapter 5. Several others helped me (often led me) in developing the empirical research discussed in chapter 5; namely, Jon Baron, Mike DeKay, Jack Hershey, Mark Kamlet, George Loewenstein, Dennis Scanlon, and Marc Spranca. Several people were kind enough to read large portions of this manuscript. Some even slugged their way through the entire thing. I am extremely grateful to Andrea Gurmankin, Michael Green, Leonard Fleck, Jon Baron, George Loewenstein, and Roy Eidelson. Ellen Wise deserves many thanks for all the patience she exhibited in working with me on this manuscript, as well as in designing many of the survey studies I present.

I could not have completed this book or the empirical research it contains without the generous support of the following: Department of Veterans Affairs, National Institutes of Health, Robert Wood Johnson Foundation, University of Pennsylvania Cancer Center, University of Pennsylvania Research Foundation, Greenwall Foundation, Rockefeller Foundation, and Department of Medicine and Center for Bioethics at the University of Pennsylvania School of Medicine.

Of course I am grateful to the people at MIT Press who helped me develop this book. Glenn McGee and Art Caplan are not only the editors for this exciting new bioethics series, they also resided in offices down the hall from me as I wrote the book. Long before I knew that they were series editors, they were helping me think about how to prepare a book proposal and how to develop a text that would broaden the audience for important bioethics issues such as those that follow. I am extremely grateful to Betty Stanton for helping me develop this book, and to all the other people at MIT Press for doing what they can to get it out to the broadest audience possible.

Finally, I have several family members who I cannot thank enough for their help. I am grateful to my parents for possibly being the first people to be excited about the idea of my writing this book; to Paula, my wife, for giving me a very powerful incentive to finish most of the writing within nine months; and to Jordan Ubel Greeno for being born right on time and for helping me think through what it really means to talk about the pricelessness of life.

Introduction

It is easy for me to retrace the course of my career and the genesis of this book and conclude that my life was preordained and this book was inevitable. In retrospect, I was destined to become a physician my freshman year of high school, when a piano teacher at the University of Minnesota said, "Peter, I will take you on as a student as long as you promise to become a physician." I had no choice but to become an ethicist when my freshman-year philosophy professor (who critiqued students' papers using a cassette recorder), after dismantling my paper for thirty minutes said, "Peter, despite all my criticisms of your paper (pause), and I take none of them back (pause), you show *some* philosophical promise." And, this book became inevitable during my first year of internal medicine residency after I read a cost-effectiveness analysis by David Eddy in which he had the effrontery to conclude that annual Papanicolaou smears were an unaffordable luxury.

In his provocative article, Eddy (1990) presented an elaborate mathematical model estimating the cost-effectiveness of Pap smears. These inexpensive tests save women's lives by detecting cervical cancer or precancerous lesions at a curable stage. Since becoming routine, annual Pap smears have significantly decreased deaths from cervical cancer.

Undeterred by the proved efficacy of these tests, Eddy and his mathematical model suggested that they were unaffordable because almost every cancer they detect would have also been detected by screening every three years. More specifically, in women who have had three normal Pap smears in the past, doing the test every three years detects 90% of cervical cancers and doing it every year detects 91%. Given the rarity of cervical cancer in this group of women, it would take $1 million of yearly Pap smears to find a single curable cervical cancer that would not have been detected by screening every three years.

Eddy's article had me totally confused. To begin with, it took me a while to understand how it could cost $1 million to save a woman's life with such an inexpensive and effective test. (The reason is that you have to test thousands of women yearly to save one life that would not have been saved by testing every three years.) But the surprising expense of yearly Pap smears was only the beginning of my confusion. I was also confused about why the *Annals of Internal Medicine,* a prominent clinical journal read by practicing physicians, would publish Eddy's article. I had been taught that physicians are not supposed to think about costs of care, but only about doing what is best for their patients. I could understand why this article might be published in a health policy or managed care journal, but what was it doing in the *Annals of Internal Medicine?* Should the cost-effectiveness of Pap smears play a role in determining what is appropriate for physicians to offer their patients? Or should it affect only insurance company and government reimbursement policies? Finally, I was confused because the article, indeed the whole enterprise of cost-effectiveness analysis, was based on the premise that life has a price, and that some life-saving interventions may not be worth their cost. But what price for life? Is $1 million too much to spend to save a life? If not, what about $2 million, $10 million, or $100 million?

The questions raised by the article, and by cost-effectiveness in general, have plagued me ever since. Clearly, there is a price that is too high to pay to prevent someone from dying of cancer. But who sets that price? And when we save money by doing Pap smears less often, what happens to the money we save? Does it simply augment some insurance company executive's annual bonus? And finally, when we decide not to offer women Pap smears every year (or every six months, or every three months), are we rationing health care?

Most of the rationing controversies I discuss in this book were staring back at me from Eddy's article.

In medical school, no one taught me anything about rationing. Nor was I taught anything about cost-effectiveness analysis—how to measure it, how to interpret it, or how to use it at the bedside. As a resident, I was seldom required to think about costs. I was told that people come to the Mayo Clinic as a last attempt to cure what ails them. Never mind that I was told the same thing at the University of Minnesota when I was in medical school and at every medical school I have worked for since. Most physicians spend medical school and residency at tertiary care (now quaternary care!) medical centers that proudly think of themselves as the health care stops of last resort. Physicians are trained to do what is best for their patients, to run every test that could find a rare, exotic disease, what in the trade is called "fascinoma," to make sure they do not miss something that another medical center, or another physician, will find. Consequently, few physicians are taught to think about costs when caring for their patients. And if they are taught anything about rationing, they are taught that it is impermissible.

Rationing has been an easy topic for medical schools and residency programs to ignore. Except for rare shortages, such as the persistent scarcity of solid organs for transplantation, those of us lucky enough to grow up in industrialized countries, with good health care systems, have not had to think much about health care rationing. When my father began practicing medicine in the 1950s and 1960s, he had a handful of antibiotics and two or three blood pressure medicines to offer his patients; the most expensive diagnostic tests available were plain-film radiographs. Computerized tomographic (CT) scans and magnetic resonance imaging (MRI) were decades away. It was easy for my father to give his patients the best health care money could buy, because there simply was not very much health care to buy.

But now, a single MRI scan, costing a couple thousand dollars, may have only a small chance of finding anything worth looking for. Intravenous immune globulin to prevent infections in patients with leukemia costs over $7 million per year of life saved (Weeks, Tierney, & Weinstein 1991). Screening for stomach cancers with fiberoptic scopes costs $420,000 per year of life saved (Read, Pass, & Komaroff 1982). Screening people six times for colon cancer with an inexpensive screening test costs over $26 million per life saved, compared with screening them only five times (Neuhauser & Lewicki 1976). Many similarly expensive tests are available that have not been proved to bring *any* kind of medical benefit. Health care is riddled with expensive, sometimes unproved toys for physicians to play with and for patients to demand.

Given the recent plethora of expensive new technologies that offer small benefits at high costs, the need to ration health care is a relatively new phenomenon. Perhaps for that reason, people are not used to the idea. Consequently, many debates on the subject dissolve into criticisms about evil governments or greedy managed care organizations rather than into honest discussions about the necessity of health care rationing. For example, in the spring of 1997 David Asch and I wrote an article in the *New England Journal of Medicine* arguing that health care rationing is ubiquitous, but is often so subtle that physicians do not even recognize that they are doing it. But no one seemed to think the article was about rationing. Instead, I heard people refer to our "article on managed care." Even Jerome Kassirer, editor of the *New England Journal*, responded with an editorial on the evils of managed care (Kassirer 1997). I went back and reread the article and found that, buried in the middle, the phrase "managed care" occurred only once. Nevertheless, to many Americans, health care rationing exists because of managed care; thus, an article about rationing was interpreted as really being about managed care. Indeed, sometimes it seems that managed care is a code word Americans use to represent everything that is wrong with the current health care system.

In the United States, people frequently debate the pros and cons of managed care organizations and whether medicine should be a for-profit business. They almost never debate health care rationing. Instead, they mention it only to accuse managed care organizations or for-profit insurance companies of some egregious crime against humanity. Clearly, there are many important issues to debate about managed care organizations and about the rampant corporatization of American health care. But these debates miss the larger issue of the need to ration health care.

Managed care organizations did not create health care rationing. Instead, the need to ration created managed care. In the United States, managed care organizations proliferated largely because of their presumed ability to contain costs. But governments in Europe, Asia, and other parts of North America are also desperate to control health care costs. Outside the United States, the need to ration health care forced governments to devise other ways besides managed care to contain costs. In Canada, patients wait for months for heart bypass surgery, only to be bumped to the back of the line when another patient becomes urgently ill (Naylor 1991). Indeed, even in the United States, managed care organizations are not the only groups engaged in rationing. Traditional fee-for-service insurance companies hire hordes of utilization reviewers to have patients discharged from the hospital earlier. State governments change eligibility criteria for Medicaid. Hospitals close down trauma centers to avoid uninsured patients. Rationing is ubiquitous. Managed care is not.

Of course, it is easier for people to argue about greedy managed care organizations, evil insurance companies, and incompetent government bureaucrats than to discuss the need to ration health care. After all, everyone agrees that managed care organizations exist. No one agrees whether rationing exists or has to exist. Instead, to many people concerned about health care cost containment, rationing is an unjustifiable evil. It is wrong that it exists. It is immoral that physicians are allowing it to occur. It is even more evil that physicians are often the ones *doing* the rationing.

Given the relatively recent push to contain health care costs, it should be no surprise that the "R" word is controversial, or that it is often used to discredit political opponents or industry competitors. "Rationing" has become a code word for immoral, inappropriate, or greedy. In fact, when a group of ethicists was recruited to help President Clinton reform the health care system (remember those days?!), they were specifically directed to draft a statement of ethical principles that did not include the word. Polls showed that the American public was against health care rationing: contain costs all you want, lower my taxes as much as you can, but don't talk about health care rationing!

Because it is so unpopular, most debates focus more on *whether* we should ration health care than on *how* we should do it. In many cases the debaters do not even agree on what it means. For example, I was once approached by a colleague who was upset about an article in which I wrote that it is sometimes morally acceptable for physicians to ration health care (Ubel & Arnold 1995a). Two weeks later, this colleague admitted one of his patients to the hospital because of an allergic reaction to a radiologic contrast dye, a solution injected into the veins to enable radiologists to visualize blood vessels and other important structures. I happened to be the attending physician on the hospital service at the time. After the patient completely recovered from the allergic reaction, I asked my colleague why he had used a standard contrast dye rather than a newer, more expensive one that would have been less likely to cause a reaction (Barret et al. 1992; Steinberg et al. 1992).

"It was appropriate to use a standard contrast dye, because this patient had no history of allergies," he replied.

I pointed out that even in such patients the newer contrast dyes are *still* less likely to cause allergic reactions than standard ones.

"That may be true," he said, "but the new dyes are simply too expensive to use on everybody."

When I asked how he could argue against health care rationing while giving this patient an inferior contrast dye, he said, "The vast majority of patients tolerate standard contrast dyes without any complications."

After more discussion, it became clear that we agreed that it was appropriate to use standard contrast dye in patients such as his because the risk of severe side effects was extremely low, but disagreed about whether this constituted rationing. I thought it was a justifiable example of rationing, and he thought it was an example of appropriate medical care. Without a clear definition, it is impossible to have a useful debate on the matter.

I want to convince people that rationing is necessary. I expect this view will be unpopular. But I am not running for public office, so the only people I have to be popular with are my wife (who is blindly in love with me) and the members of my tenure review board (who won't read this book). I can afford to be unpopular.

We cannot have it all. We cannot afford to give every health service to every person who could possibly benefit. Most people's health would improve if they had dietitians review what they ate for dinner and physical therapists work the kinks out of their lower backs. Most hospitalized patients and most nursing home residents would benefit from a higher nurse-to-patient ratio. If we could really afford to have it all, standard contrast dyes would no longer be standard, and newer, more expensive dyes would be offered to everyone. If every beneficial health care service was affordable, we would not need people like David Eddy to conduct cost-effectiveness analyses. Instead, we would only concern ourselves with *effectiveness* analyses—showing us what works best so we could make sure everyone gets it. But there are limits to what we can offer everyone, and we must start figuring out how to set those limits.

In traveling farther down this road of gloom and doom, I am not only going to insist that we have to ration health care, but also that some of this rationing ought to be done by physicians at the bedside, and that our most useful rationing tool (at the bedside and at policy levels) is cost-effectiveness analysis. Although there are ethical problems with physicians rationing from their patients, and with rationing according to cost-effectiveness, bedside rationing, based on cost-effectiveness, ought to play a larger role.

The moral questions raised by cost-effectiveness analysis deserve to be debated by a broad audience. In this book, I attempt to present a general overview of moral and methodological controversies raised by cost-effectiveness analysis, especially with regard to its role as a guide for how to ration health care. In doing so, I do not go into the kind of economic depth an economist would prefer and I do not pursue each theory with the rigor a philosopher would expect. Although depth and rigor are important, it is also important to draw people into the debates who might otherwise stand on the sidelines. In addition, sometimes depth and rigor have to be relaxed in order to pull together insights across a number of disciplines. I have written a book that mixes ethical arguments about the appropriate role of cost-effectiveness in health care rationing, with empirical research about how the general public wants to ration health care, with clinical insights I have gained through my practice of general internal medicine. By straddling the disciplines of ethics, economics, research psychology, and clinical medicine, I hope to draw new people into continuing debates about the appropriate role of cost-effectiveness analysis in guiding health care rationing decisions.

This book is not the final word on health care rationing or on cost-effectiveness analysis. Many issues have to be worked out so that we can ration more ethically. But I hope this book will advance the debates so we can focus more on *how* to ration rather than remaining bogged down in debates about *whether* to do it. Life has immense value, but it also has a price. We must decide how much we want to spend on health care to extend and improve our lives.

I

Cost-Effectiveness and the Controversial Necessity of Health Care Rationing

1

Rationing According to Cost-Effectiveness: Explicit, Quantifiable, and Unacceptable?

It may have started out with a touch of fatigue, but soon it was clear that something was dramatically wrong with Coby Howard. The seven-year-old boy was seriously ill; fatally ill, it turned out. Coby had acute leukemia. Chemotherapy alone could not halt the proliferation of his cancerous white blood cells. Coby was dying, and bone marrow transplantation was his only chance of survival.

But Coby did not come from money, and Oregon's Medicaid program refused to pay for a bone marrow transplant. The year was 1987, and Oregon had stopped paying for Medicaid transplants in order to increase the number of people eligible for its program (Welch & Larson 1988). The state estimated that thirty-four Medicaid enrollees would require transplants in the upcoming year. Given the huge expense of these procedures, the money Oregon would save by halting this funding could be used to provide basic health care coverage to 1500 new enrollees. Thirty-four unidentifiable, "statistical lives" seemed like a small price to pay to provide 1500 people with basic health care.

Enter Coby Howard. The media picked up his tragic story, and the thirty-four previously unidentifiable lives now bore the highly identifiable and cute face of this desperate boy. The public was outraged and the legislature was embarrassed. Soon the state reinstituted transplant funding, and found additional money to keep paying for the 1500 new Medicaid enrollees. Unfortunately, these legislative changes did not occur quickly enough to save Coby's life.

With the benefit of hindsight, it is easy to criticize Oregon's decision to halt transplant funding. After all, how could anyone think that the public would stand by and watch helpless children die merely because the state was too cheap to pay for a transplant? But the Oregon legislature should not be condemned so quickly. Even now, more than a decade after this debacle, few legislators in any U.S. state are willing to acknowledge the need to ration health care. Yet, here they were in 1987, during the economic boom of Reagan's presidency, willing to acknowledge explicitly not only the need to ration, but also the grim realities of trying to provide basic health care for poor people in the face of hyperinflationary tertiary care medicine. Whereas Oregon's legislators exercised questionable judgment by deciding to halt Medicaid transplant funding, their decision was motivated by brave and honorable intentions; they truly desired to maximize the health benefits the state could provide to its Medicaid enrollees.

Despite intense criticism of how it had handled the Coby Howard "situation," the legislators did not give up in their efforts to change Oregon's Medicaid program. When the sorry business ended, they went back to the drawing board and tried to figure out if there were better ways of saving money than halting transplant funding. Although transplants were incredibly expensive in 1987, for many people they were also life saving. Why pick on these procedures, the legislature reasoned, when slightly less expensive health care services might bring significantly smaller benefits? In fact, some services might even bring no benefit and cost a fair amount of money! Oregon turned to cost-effectiveness analysis (Kitzhaber 1993).

The plan was simple. The legislature appointed a commission and gave it the job of ranking Medicaid services from most to least cost effective. Services that bring large benefits at small cost would be at the top of the list, and those that bring few benefits at high cost would be at the bottom. The state would then estimate the cost of providing each service to an expanded number of Medicaid beneficiaries, starting at the top of the list and moving down until the money ran out. At that point, it would draw a line and all services below the line, the least cost-effective ones, would no longer be reimbursed by the Medicaid program (Oregon Health Services Commission 1991). By refusing to pay for services that are not very cost effective, the state would save money, enabling it to add extra people to Medicaid.

This plan was a textbook example of how many people think cost-effectiveness analysis (CEA) should be used to ration health care (Eddy

1991b; Kaplan 1992). CEA shows how to maximize health benefits within a specific health care budget. By specifying its Medicaid budget and the number of people that would be covered, Oregon could determine which services it could afford. Thus it would in theory show how to buy the greatest amount of medical benefit with its Medicaid dollars.

This was a bold and ambitious plan—bold for admitting the need to ration health care, and ambitious for trying to determine the cost-effectiveness of a huge number of health care services at a time when the medical literature was not exactly overflowing with cost-effectiveness studies. The plan was hotly debated. Many were enthusiastic that Oregon was explicitly admitting the need to ration health care. But many others questioned whether it was fair to conduct such a huge social experiment on a Medicaid population (Daniels 1992) and were skeptical of intentions to extend the rationing scheme to all of the state's citizens.

Why Turn to Cost-Effectiveness Analysis?

Cost-effectiveness analysis seemed like an ideal tool to help Oregon identify ways to save money on Medicaid services so it could provide benefits to more people. In theory, CEA enables policy planners to compare how much benefit patients are receiving from seemingly incomparable health care services (Eddy 1992b; Gold et al. 1996). If a moderately expensive treatment brings large benefits, CEA can show whether it is more cost effective than a slightly expensive treatment that brings moderate benefits. In addition, CEA can even compare the cost-effectiveness of life-saving treatments and over-the-counter remedies for the common cold. (Later, I explain how CEA allows us to compare the seemingly incomparable.)

Cost-effectiveness information has a powerful ability to influence thinking about health care rationing. Decisions about whether women should have yearly Pap smears, for example, are fundamentally altered by information that the additional cost per cervical cancer detected compared with every three years is over $1 million (Eddy, 1990). Putting a dollar value on human life is a stark, dramatic, and explicit way to shape thinking about how much we value certain health care services. Are we prepared to spend $1 million for every cervical cancer that we detect? If so, are we equally willing to spend money on other services that cost $1 million for every life that they save? What if there are thousands of such interventions? Are we willing to spend thousands of millions of dollars in such a way? It is nearly impossible to imagine a debate about the social merits of offering Pap smears every year versus every three years without considering cost-effectiveness.

Cost-effectiveness information often highlights the counterintuitively high expense of some seemingly inexpensive medical services. Imagine we offer a $20 screening test to a group of 2,000 people at a total cost of $2 million. The test saves 100 lives, at a cost of $20,000 per life saved. This seems like a bargain. What society would not want to spend $20,000 to save someone's life, or $2 million to save 100 lives? But what if an alternative screening test was available that was half as expensive and would save ninety-nine lives? According to CEA, the existence of this less expensive test radically alters the cost-effectiveness of the first test. As we have seen, the first test costs $2 million; the alternative test costs only $1 million. The first test saves 100 lives and the second saves 99. Thus, the real cost-effectiveness of the first test is not $20,000 per life saved, but $1 million per life saved. We have to increase spending from $1 million to $2 million to save one additional life.

Whatever you think about the value of life, spending $1 million to prevent a fatal disease is a very different prospect than spending $20,000. Cost-effective analysis can show us how much we really have to spend on specific health care services to bring specific health care benefits.

Cost-effectiveness analysis does not tell policy planners how much money they should spend to save a life. Instead, it provides information to inform allocation decisions. Its power lies in its ability to provide explicit information that focuses decision making about how to set health care priorities.

It makes allocation trade-offs explicit. If a health insurance company reimburses for Pap smears every three years instead of yearly, CEA can estimate how much money it will save and how many enrollees' lives will be lost. If a radiology department is deciding whether to purchase a new mammography machine or spend more money on safer contrast dyes, CEA can show the costs and benefits of each purchasing option. And, if Oregon's Medicaid program wanted to find out how to expand enrollment criteria while keeping within its budget constraints, CEA could show which medical services could be abandoned with the least detriment to people's health.

Thus CEA is informative, explicit, and quantitative, traits that recommend it as a rationing tool. But it is not merely a dry, mathematical combination of medical outcome statistics. Rather, it purports to capture public values in its measurements. It is two pinches of scientific data with one teaspoon of community values. It not only provides information about how much money it costs to bring certain health care benefits, but also incorporates a measure of community values, utility measurement, that attempts to reveal the relative importance the general public places on these benefits (Torrance 1986). If CEA only told us that it cost $100 to cure a plantar wart and $50,000 to prevent a heart attack, we would not be much better off than when we started. We would still have to decide the relative importance of curing plantar warts versus preventing heart attacks. By measuring health-related utility, CEA purports to show the relative importance of various health benefits.

To illustrate how CEA attempts to capture community values for how to ration health care, and to show how it is supposed to guide health care allocation decisions, it is time to return to Oregon to see how it planned to ration Medicaid services.

Making Oregon's Cost-Effectiveness List

After deciding to ration according to cost-effectiveness, the Oregon legislature appointed a commission with the task of creating a cost-effectiveness list. The commission scoured the medical literature to gather data, but cost-effectiveness studies were scant, and the commission ultimately had to rely on expert panels to estimate the costs and effectiveness of various services (Oregon Health Services Commission 1991). Lung specialists, for example, were asked to estimate the costs and effectiveness of treating pneumonia.

The commission also had to estimate the relative value its citizens placed on various health outcomes. If lung specialists concluded, for example, that it costs an average of $50,000 to save the life of a patient with pneumonia and $20,000 to give palliative therapy to someone dying of incurable lung cancer, society must have some way to judge the relative benefits of life-saving pneumonia treatments and palliative care. Health care services, after all, do a wide range of things. Some offer treatments for plantar warts. Others provide relief of symptoms of chronic pain or congestive heart failure. Yet others potentially save people's lives. To estimate the relative cost-effectiveness of these incredibly varied services, CEA requires some common unit of measurement to help compare them.

That common unit of measurement is called a quality-adjusted life-year, or QALY (pronounced "qualy"). To help measure QALYs, the Oregon commission conducted a telephone survey of 1,000 randomly selected Oregonians and asked questions such as the following:

Imagine your legs are paralyzed and you can not walk; you must use a wheelchair to get around. Otherwise you are healthy. On a scale from zero (for conditions as bad as death) to 100 (for perfect health), with 50 halfway in between, how would you rate the condition?

People's responses to these questions were used to determine the relative benefits of various health care interventions. Imagine two health conditions, one with a value of 50 on this 100-point scale, and another with a value of 75. Curing the former brings 50 points of benefit (an improvement from 50 to 100 on the scale) and curing the latter brings 25. The Oregon list makers assumed the 100-point scale was an interval scale, like a temperature scale, in which equal changes in the value of a health condition are equally important to achieve, and in which a change that is twice as large as another change brings twice the benefit. An improvement in health from a condition with a rating of 50 to a condition with a rating of 75 brings the same amount of benefit as improving a condition from 75 to 100, and an improvement from 50 to 100 is twice as beneficial as an improvement from 75 to 100. (In a similar manner, an increase in temperature from 10 to 20 degrees is half as large as a change from 10 to 30 degrees, and also half as large as a change from 70 to 90 degrees.)

Measures such as the 100-point rating scale are commonly employed in CEAs to estimate the number of QALYs brought by health care interventions (Loomes & McKenzie 1989). An intervention that extends a person's life for one year and provides perfect health generates one QALY. In contrast, an intervention that extends a person's life for one year but at a diminished quality of life, with a value of 50, produces half as much benefit, or 0.5 QALYs. An intervention that does not extend a person's life, but improves quality of life from 50 to 75 produces 0.25 QALYs per year.

Once the commission estimated the cost of all the interventions, the medical benefits they brought, and the relative value people place on them, it could determine their cost-effectiveness and rank them from most to least cost effective. With the help of a team of actuaries, it could estimate the cost of offering each of these health care services to Medicaid enrollees. Starting at the top of the list, Oregon could offer services to enrollees, moving down the list to the point at which the actuaries estimated it would run out of funds. At that point, the state could draw a line across the list above which services would be provided to all Medicaid enrollees and below which services would be unavailable to them all.

The cost-effectiveness list was finally complete—and it was a complete failure. The commission did not even forward it to the legislature. The members concluded that it did not capture peoples' values for how to set health care priorities (Hadorn 1991). A now infamous example illustrates the commission's reluctance: the list ranked splints for temporomandibular joint (TMJ) pain as being more cost effective (and thus more important) than treatment of acutely fatal appendicitis (Eddy 1991b). How could TMJ splints be more cost-effective than saving people's life with a simple operation?

What Happened in Oregon?

What happened in Oregon? Why did its cost-effectiveness list fail so miserably?

Much of this book is an attempt to explore the failure of cost-effectiveness to capture public rationing preferences in ways useful for setting health care priorities. Clearly, Oregon's cost-effectiveness list had a billion problems. As stated above, Oregon had almost no published cost-effectiveness analyses to help it make its ranking. Consequently, the data it used to estimate cost effectiveness were suspect at best. And the measurement methods, some of which I discuss in more detail later, were controversial, raising questions about whether it had even used the appropriate techniques to make its list.

But much more was going on in Oregon than can be blamed on faulty data or questionable measurement techniques. Instead, the rejection of the list as a priority-setting tool resulted from a wide array of moral controversies which Oregonians had not adequately sorted out. And Oregonians, it should be added, are farther along in thinking about the need to ration health care than are most Americans. In fact, it was the peculiar wonderfulness of the state that even allowed its citizens to acknowledge explicitly the need to ration health care and to set out to try to improve access to Medicaid.

We have only recently entered an era in which some health care services, even though they bring important benefits, may be unaffordable. And we have yet to agree on how society, through government, third-party payers, or health care providers, ought to ration health care.

Oregon's efforts raise fundamental questions that deserve our attention. Did the cost-effectiveness list fail because the public rejected any attempt to ration health care from vulnerable Medicaid enrollees? Or did it fail because it *explicitly* rationed services from Medicaid enrollees? Was cost-effectiveness at fault for the failure? What moral assumptions does cost-effectiveness make about how we ought to ration health care? And are these assumptions acceptable? Did Oregon's list fail for the same reason any government rationing plan will fail—health care is simply too complex to rely on a government rationing list to make these decisions? Should Oregon have relied on clinicians to make these decisions, people who could take account of clinical complexities that could not be captured in its ranking?

There are more than enough questions and controversies to fill this book, and many of them cannot be successfully answered or resolved. Although CEA is a powerful tool to guide health care rationing decisions, it is an imperfect one. At most, it should be used only to guide such decisions.

But I am getting ahead of myself. Before judging the strengths and weaknesses of CEA, I must look more closely at whether any types of rationing decisions are necessary and at what debates tell us about the appropriate role of cost-effectiveness in guiding those decisions.

2
The Politics of Defining Health Care Rationing

A while back I was asked by a national medical organization to comment on a policy paper it had drafted, in which it maintained that governments, physicians, and third-party payers should never ration medical care. To make this statement, the organization defined rationing, from what I could tell, so that all actions it thought were *inappropriate* would be examples of rationing, and those actions it thought were *appropriate* would be examples of something else. For instance, the organization stated that Oregon's Medicaid initiative that proposed to increase the number of Medicaid enrollees by limiting the number of health services offered was not an example of health care rationing, but was instead an example of "appropriate health care priority setting." Yet this plan was almost universally described by proponents and opponents as the Oregon rationing plan (Daniels 1991; Fox & Leichter 1991; Garland 1992).

Which is it? Was Oregon's list a government-sponsored rationing plan, or was it an example of appropriate health care priority setting? Does it even matter whether this priority-setting exercise qualified as "rationing"?

Despite consensus among most experts that health care costs must be contained, great controversy surrounds whether it is ever acceptable to ration health care. Part of this controversy results from disagreement about whether costs can be adequately contained by eliminating waste rather than by rationing. But controversy also arises from disagreements about what it means to ration health care. Earlier I described a tortuous (and even torturous) conversation with a colleague about whether using standard contrast dye for a patient receiving a radiology test was an example of rationing. As with many debates I have encountered over the years, it took a while for both of us to realize that we had very different ideas about the entire concept.

The medical literature contains numerous casual and formal definitions of rationing. A sample will suffice to show the range of meanings people place on these words. Some experts state that health care rationing involves an "inequitable distribution of resources based on inability to pay" (Hadorn & Brook 1991). Others define it as "the equitable distribution of scarce resources" (Churchill 1987), as the "denial of commodities to those who have the money to buy them" (Aaron & Schwartz 1990), "the deliberate and systematic denial of certain kinds of services, even when they are known to be beneficial because they are deemed to be too expensive" (Relman 1990a), and "any set of activities that determines who gets needed medical care when resources are insufficient to provide for all" (Brook & Lohr 1986).

It should be no surprise that the term encompasses such a dizzying array of definitions. Nor should it be surprising that so many experts state strong positions about the appropriateness or inappropriateness, evilness or saintliness, of health care rationing without even clarifying what they mean. That is how language works. We have a general idea of what most words mean, until we try to pin them down. Then we find that we have never been all that clear about exactly what we are talking about.

In my first college philosophy class (which my parents say ruined me, but which I think made it obvious that I was already ruined), we were asked to read a Platonic dialogue, *The Meno,* named after a man unfortunate enough to be caught in a debate with Socrates about whether virtue is something that can be taught. Little does poor, unsuspecting Meno realize that rather than answering this question, Socrates will show him that he has no idea what virtue is: "we shall not understand the truth of the matter until, before asking how men get virtue, we try to discover what virtue is in and of itself" (Hamilton & Cairns 1961). After an exhausting discussion in which Meno is forced to acknowledge that he has no idea what virtue is, Socrates says that he's late for a date, gotta go (my translation), and walks away leaving Meno to ponder how much less he understood about the world than he thought he did moments before. (The reader is consoled only by the knowledge that Socrates thinks awareness of one's ignorance is a sign of great knowledge.)

I have repeated Meno's mistake many times, not by getting caught in a debate with Socrates (I wish!), but by trying to pin down the un-pin-downable. Rationing is a word, and it is up to us to decide how we want to use it. It has no single "correct" meaning. Health care rationing has, and will continue to have, many different definitions.

Disagreements about what it means inform our understanding of Oregon's experiences. Indeed, debates about the appropriateness or inappropriateness of any kind of rationing scheme must be viewed within the context of the particular definition being espoused. Therefore, in this chapter, I review three distinguishing characteristics of these definitions and show what they tell us about the failure of Oregon's cost-effectiveness list and about the politics of debating the appropriateness of health care rationing.

Three Distinguishing Characteristics of Rationing Definitions

The confusing array of definitions listed above reflects different notions of what constitutes health care rationing. The definitions differ from each other in at least three ways. First, they differ according to whether something has to be *explicit* to qualify as rationing. Some hold that rationing includes only conscious decisions taken at an administrative level that make a service unavailable to some people (Brook & Lohr 1986). In contrast, others say that nonexplicit mechanisms, such as allocating goods by the free market, also qualify as rationing (Hall 1994). Second, definitions differ according to whether a resource must be *absolutely scarce* before its distribution qualifies as rationing. Some people think rationing is limited to the distribution of absolutely scarce resources, such as transplantable organs (Evans 1983), whereas others think it can also refer to allocation of nonscarce resources, such as access to subspecialists and prescriptions for expensive medicines (Hall 1997). Third, they differ according to whether rationing only involves limits on *necessary* services, such as dialysis for patients with end-stage renal disease (Hadorn & Brook 1991; Relman 1990a) or whether limits on

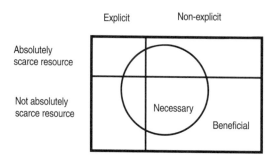

Figure 2.1
Three distinctions among rationing definitions.

any *beneficial* but unnecessary services also qualify as rationing (Hall 1997; Mechanic 1979; Ubel & Arnold 1995a; Ubel & Goold 1997a).

Figure 2.1 illustrates these three distinctions among rationing definitions. In this figure, the vertical line separates medical services that are limited explicitly versus those that are limited nonexplicitly. This line is to the left of the midpoint to suggest that more services are withheld nonexplicitly than explicitly, although the exact ratio is not represented. The horizontal line separates absolutely scarce resources from those that are not absolutely scarce. The horizontal line is above the midpoint of the diagram to suggest that few resources are absolutely scarce, although the exact ratio of scarce to nonscarce resources is not represented. Finally, within the figure is a circle. Inside the circle are health care services thought to be necessary; outside the circle are those that are thought to be beneficial, but not necessary.

The figure is helpful in illustrating differences among definitions of health care rationing. For example, the view that rationing involves only the explicit distribution of absolutely scarce and necessary resources, such as life-saving transplants, is represented by the shaded part of figure 2.2. A slightly less restrictive view, that rationing includes the explicit distribution of absolutely scarce resources that are either necessary or beneficial, is represented by the shaded regions of figure 2.3. And the view of most health care economists, that health care rationing is any implicit or explicit mechanism that allows people to go without beneficial services, is reproduced in figure 2.4 (Fuchs 1984; Hall 1997; Mechanic 1992; Orentlicher 1994; Reinhardt 1997).

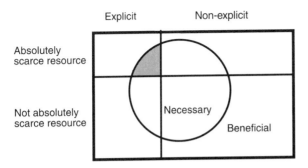

Figure 2.2
Rationing is the explicit distribution of absolutely scarce, necessary resources.

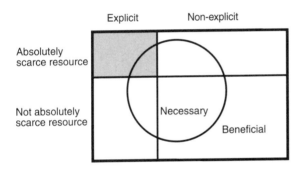

Figure 2.3
Rationing is the explicit distribution of absolutely scarce, beneficial resources.

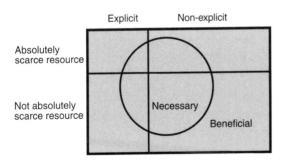

Figure 2.4
Rationing is any mechanism allowing people to go without beneficial health care.

Tangled somewhere among these confusing linguistic threads are crucial issues. None of these definitions is neutral. Each carries emotional and political contents that are often used to influence debates about the appropriateness or inappropriateness of particular health care policies. Indeed, rationing has become such a loaded phrase that debates about its meaning often hinge on whether those defining it want to support or condemn a specific policy, much like the national medical organization described above that made great efforts to define rationing in a way that would exclude Oregon's Medicaid plan in order to show its support of the plan.

The Danger of Limiting Health Care Rationing to Explicit Mechanisms

Bill H. had been running a small business for over twenty years. His ten employees put up with his quick temper and erratic behavior because they knew deep down he was a true friend who would do anything he could to help them out in times of need. But they were unaware that Bill's erratic behavior was due in part to the fact that he was an alcoholic, a long-term alcoholic. Through years of heavy drinking Bill's liver had shriveled up to a knobby shadow of its former self. Bill needed a liver transplant.

But Bill could not stop drinking. Three stays in an expensive rehabilitation center, and the support of family and friends, were not enough to make him stop. And because he continued to drink no transplant team in the country was willing to give him a new liver.

Most liver transplant centers refuse organs for patients with alcoholic cirrhosis who continue to drink alcohol. In fact, many insurance companies in the United States refuse to pay for liver transplants in actively drinking alcoholics. In short, livers are *explicitly* rationed from alcoholics until these patients convince a transplant team that they have stopped drinking.

Few would question whether an explicit policy such as this is an example of rationing. But is such an explicit policy the only type of action that qualifies as health care rationing? If liver transplants or other health care services are implicitly withheld from patients, is this any less of an example of rationing?

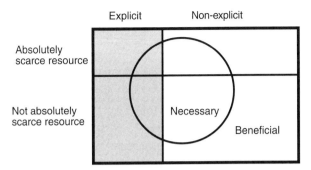

Figure 2.5
Limiting health care rationing to explicit mechanisms.

As mentioned, some people define rationing as the explicit denial of health care services to people who could benefit from them (Havighurst 1992). By this view, it involves explicit decisions about how many and what types of health care goods people will receive (see figure 2.5). This definition is reminiscent of U.S. government practices during World War II, when it limited the amount of gasoline and aluminum foil that people could buy.

It is important to understand that, according to this definition, the explicit denial of health care services is not merely an example of rationing, but it is the *only* example of rationing. That is, for something to qualify as rationing, it must involve explicit denial of health care services to people who could benefit from them.

According to this definition, limiting the availability of health care services by ability to pay is not an example of explicit rationing. In contrast, economists view ability to pay as a rationing mechanism. To them, rationing includes any mechanisms that limit how many goods people receive, including willingness to pay. Society rations BMWs by requiring people to pay for them. Similarly, it could ration MRIs by ability to pay. To an economist, this would involve rationing, even though no one explicitly decided to limit the number of MRIs or decided which particular people would have them.

To many people, the economic definition of rationing will seem out of sorts with popular understanding of the term. After all, people do not generally think that BMWs are rationed. If common usage were determining the best definition of health care rationing, the explicit view would seem to win out over the economists' broader view. However, people do not think about health care the way they think about automobiles or videocassette recorders. Suppose that Bill H. stopped drinking a year ago, after his company went bankrupt. He turned his life around and was even reunited with his wife. But he could no longer afford health insurance. Too wealthy to qualify for Medicaid, too young to qualify for Medicare, and too poor to afford health insurance, Bill was doomed to die of liver failure because no transplant center was willing to give him a transplant unless he could come up with the money.

People think that many health care services are necessary and vitally important in a way that BMWs and videocassette recorders are not. Allowing someone to go without a liver transplant because he does not have enough money would strike most people as paradigmatic of health care rationing. Indeed, Coby Howard, the seven-year-old with leukemia, was not forbidden from receiving a bone marrow transplant. The state simply refused to *pay* for it. If Coby's family had been able to come up with the money, he would have received the transplant. My point is that many health care services, probably most of them, if distributed purely on the basis of ability to pay, would strike most people as being rationed.

Although explicit programs to deny health care services are appropriately classified as rationing, we should not limit rationing to such explicit mechanisms, because some services are so important that distributing them according to ability to pay results in deprivation and hardship commonly associated with rationing. Health care is a special consumer good. It can be essential for people's ability to enjoy their lives, or even to live at all. It is often necessary so that people have fair opportunities to pursue important life goals (Daniels 1985). This is why experts debate whether we have a right to health care, but do not debate whether we have a right to VCRs, BMWs, or built-in bookcases.

In fact, it is dangerous to limit the definition of rationing so that it encompasses only explicit mechanisms: health care providers or third-party payers who want to avoid being accused of rationing will simply resort to implicit mechanisms and insist that they are not rationing (since rationing is explicit). "I wasn't rationing. I was just giving it to the person willing to pay the most!" Because explicit rationing is often morally preferable to implicit rationing, a broad definition that includes both mechanisms might decrease the chance that people in power will resort to implicit mechanisms to avoid being accused of rationing.

What does the distinction between explicit and implicit health care rationing tell us about Oregon's plan? Failure of the cost-effectiveness list can partly be blamed on its explicitness. Clearly, if the commission had devised the list and secretly distributed it to health care providers as a guideline to keep in mind when treating Medicaid patients (perhaps accompanied by a financial incentive to limit the amount of money spent on these patients), the list may have been adopted. The explicitness of this plan highlighted deficiencies in the list. Nevertheless, Oregon eventually created another rationing list (which I discuss later in this chapter). Although it was not based on cost-effectiveness, it still was based on the idea of stating that, statewide, certain explicit services would no longer be available to Medicaid enrollees. The list ultimately became law. Thus, at least in Oregon, explicitness does not doom a rationing plan.

Problems with Limiting Health Care Rationing to Absolutely Scarce Resources

Suppose Bill H. had turned his life around in time to save his liver, but not in time to save his company. He stopped drinking and his liver recovered. (The liver, in fact, has an amazing ability to recover from injury. If half of a person's liver is removed because of injury, the remaining tissue will regenerate so quickly that within six months the person will have a normal-size and normally functioning organ.) Unfortunately, the stress of his failed company took its toll and Bill had a small heart attack. Moreover, his doctors were worried that he would have a large heart attack unless he underwent bypass surgery. But bypass surgery was not in Bill's future because he no longer had health insurance. Consequently, he could not find a surgeon willing to operate on him.

Some people consider that health care rationing applies only to the distribution of absolutely scarce resources, such as transplant organs, and not of nonscarce resources (figure 2.6). For example, Roger Evans (1983) distinguished between allocation and rationing. By allocation he meant aggregate-level decisions about what types and amounts of health care

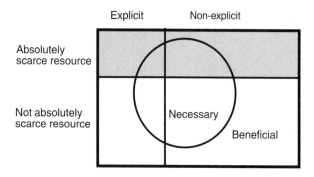

Figure 2.6
Rationing is the distribution of absolutely scarce resources.

resources to make available, such as the number of intensive care beds or MRI scanners. By rationing, in contrast, he meant "the process by which criteria are applied to selectively discriminate among patients who are eligible for resources that had been previously allocated to various programs" (Evans 1983).

By this view, rationing involves divvying up the health care pie, whereas allocation involves deciding how big to make the pie. In effect, allocation decisions limit resources. Once a resource is absolutely scarce because of an allocation decision, it can be rationed. Consequently, the lower part of figure 2.6 is not part of rationing. However, a resource that otherwise would have been available, such as an MRI scanner, is pushed into the upper part of the figure by a decision to limit its availability.

Evans's distinction between allocation and rationing is reminiscent of Calabresi and Bobbit's (1978) distinction between "first-order" and "second-order" tragic choices. They explored the painful choices that become necessary when goods are scarce. Those things that Evans called allocation decisions, such as determining how many dialysis machines to make available to patients, Calabresi and Bobbit called first-order tragic choices. And those things Evans calls rationing decisions, such as who should undergo treatment with available dialysis machines, they called second-order tragic choices.

At first glance, this discussion may seem unnecessary. You say "tomato," I say "tomahto." You say "allocation," I say "first-order tragic choice." And, indeed, the most important thing we can do is clarify our terms. Evans, Calabresi, and Bobbit should all be congratulated for defining these terms so clearly (and explicitly!). But, Calabresi and Bobbit's language can be usefully compared with Evans's. Think of the emotional impact of three terms: tragic choices, rationing, and allocation. If you were a high school student taking the SAT, which term would you say does not belong on this list? My guess is you would choose allocation because it seems out of character with the morally charged, emotionally loaded language of tragic choices and rationing. People do not engage in heated emotional debates about whether it is necessary to "allocate" health care. Politicians don't accuse other politicians of "allocating" health care.

Decisions Evans calls allocation and those he calls rationing have one thing in common—they all involve tragic choices. Calabresi and Bobbit's illuminating book reminds us of this fact. For example, decisions about who should receive dialysis treatment are tragic, because they determine who will live and die. But, decisions to limit the number of dialysis machines available are equally tragic, because they determine that not enough machines will be available to treat all the people who need the procedure. A major problem I have with Evans's distinction between allocation and rationing is that allocation is too bland a term to refer to what are often tragic decisions regarding how much of a health care resource to make available, and it simply does not have enough impact to highlight the moral significance of these decisions.

By calling both first-order and second-order decisions tragic choices, Calabresi and Bobbit highlighted the moral significance of both kinds of decisions. In addition, by lumping both types of decisions together under the rubric of tragic, they highlighted the overlap between them. The authors admitted that their distinction between first- and second-order decisions is an oversimplification.

Rationing decisions have many levels, and influence can travel from higher levels to lower levels and vice versa. Higher-level decisions generally affect more people than lower-level ones. A public policy decision to base health care on a free market has a huge effect on almost everyone, and a corresponding decision to link health insurance with employment has a large effect on unemployed people. At a lower level, a managed care organization's decision not to hire a pediatric surgeon would mainly affect children in the plan who require surgery, although it may free up more resources for other patients. At the lowest level, a decision by a doctor that a specific health care resource is not medically necessary would primarily affect the individual patient in question. But even these lowest-level decisions influence, in a small way, higher levels. The number of MRI machines available, for example, influences doctors' decisions about who will have an MRI scan, whereas doctors' collective decisions about who should have an MRI scan influence higher-level decisions about whether to purchase additional MRI machines. All of these decisions, whether implicit or explicit, whether involving absolutely or relatively scarce resources, have important implications for health care rationing. All layers involve tragic choices. Evans's distinction between allocation and rationing suggests a stronger separation than exists.

When Oregon refused to pay for Coby Howard's bone marrow transplant, it was not limiting the availability of an absolutely scarce resource. Bone marrow transplants, unlike heart, kidney, and liver transplants, do not involve an absolutely scarce resource. Kidneys and livers are usually collected from cadavers, and there is a growing shortage of organs available to those who need them. Bone marrow tissue, on the other hand, can be collected from living donors with minimal risk, and thus it is not absolutely scarce. Hence, if we consider health care rationing to refer only to the distribution of absolutely scarce resources, Coby Howard's situation would not qualify as rationing but would be an example of allocation. Clearly, Coby's situation deserves all the emotional content of phrases such as tragic choices and health care rationing. Similarly, a decision to withhold bypass surgery from Bill because he had no insurance deserves to be called rationing even though bypass surgery is not an absolutely scarce resource.

The Confusion Caused by Limiting Health Care Rationing to Withholding of Necessary Services

Poor Bill H. After struggling through liver disease, alcoholism, heart attacks, and business failure, and after being unable to have bypass surgery, he had the big one, a massive heart attack that left him with severe congestive heart failure. He could no longer walk up a flight of stairs without resting to catch his breath. Fortunately for Bill, by the time this happened his wife had found a new job that provided him with health insurance. He and his wife chose the most affordable policy offered by her employer, a managed care plan called Health Care Is Us. Health Care Is Us kept its rates low by aggressively encouraging its physicians to cut costs. In part, these cost-containment efforts, in parallel with a series of practice guidelines the company developed, succeeded in getting physicians to stop prescribing unnecessary and potentially harmful drugs and diagnostic tests. But they also convinced many clinicians, including Bill's new physician, to trim some marginally beneficial services that came at significant expense.

Bill received all the important medicine he required for his congestive heart failure, to relieve his shortness of breath and to increase his chance of survival. He received agents to lower his cholesterol and to reduce the probability of another heart attack. But his new physician was conservative in ordering screening tests to look for other diseases Bill might be developing. For example, this physician screened his patients for colon cancer with a flexible sigmoidoscope, an instrument that looks at only the last 60 centimeters of the colon. He ignored other screening tests, such as colon films, that visualize the entire colon.

Bill developed colon cancer in the proximal part of his colon, which was not visualized by flexible sigmoidoscopy, and is recovering from surgery. His tumor is no longer curable, as it might have been if another screening test had detected it earlier. The physician's decision to screen Bill with a flexible sigmoidoscope, a decision that is well within the standard of care, may have cost Bill his life.

The third distinction dividing definitions involves whether health care rationing must involve the withholding of necessary services. David Hadorn and Robert Brook, two internationally recognized experts on health care policy, define health care rationing as "the withholding of necessary services" as opposed to beneficial services that are not necessary (Hadorn & Brook 1991; figure 2.7). This contrasts with a broader, economic view that rationing involves withholding beneficial services whether or not they are necessary (Fuchs 1998). Economists view rationing as being omnipresent. It is simply any method used to distribute scarce resources, and all resources are scarce because desires are always

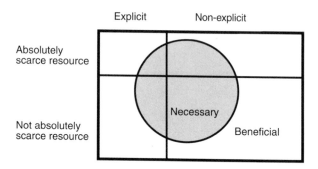

Figure 2.7
Rationing is the withholding of necessary services.

greater than the ability to fulfill them. According to economists, health care can be rationed by willingness to pay, ability to pay, insurance company administrative decisions, or government laws (Reinhardt, 1996). Anything that keeps people from obtaining every potentially beneficial medical service is a type of rationing.

Hadorn and Brook limit rationing to the withholding of *necessary* services to take advantage of the largely negative connotations associated with it. According to their view, it is rarely if ever justifiable to withhold necessary medical services.

Their definition ignores many other ethically important decisions regarding when to offer beneficial services to patients. Hadorn (1992a) proposes that a panel of scientific experts should determine which services are necessary. But such a panel potentially obscures the fact that these determinations often require value judgments. A decision regarding what to do about a promising new health care service of unproved benefit relies on a value judgment about what it means for a benefit to be unproved. Hadorn's reliance on scientific experts could camouflage important moral decisions by making them appear to be strictly scientific decisions.

To make matters worse, when expert panels make decisions about what services are necessary, they will inevitably have to decide whether certain benefits are worth their cost. What would the panel conclude about colon cancer screening? Would it be "necessary" to detect the majority of these lesions by flexible sigmoidoscopy, but unnecessary to detect the remainder with a colon film (Eddy 1990)? When does a valuable outcome such as preventing death from colon cancer become so expensive that it is no longer necessary? Decisions about whether it is necessary to have flexible sigmoidoscopies and/or colon radiographs reflect value judgments about the cost-worthiness of the two approaches. Hadorn does not deny that designing basic benefits packages requires value judgments. But determining necessity by a scientific panel makes it easy for others to misinterpret these judgments as being value neutral.

Decisions about when the costs of a medical benefit are too high to be worth while should not be linked with the word "necessary." Cost-worthiness judgments do not determine what is necessary. Moreover, the confounding of necessity and affordability confuses many people. Does the unaffordability of a life-saving technology make it any less necessary to have one's life saved? If Hadorn's expert panel is asked to make judgments about whether benefits are affordable, it should be called an affordability panel, so everyone will know what the panel is doing and can debate the value of life, liberty, and the pursuit of happiness. But if the panel is asked only to decide what health care is necessary, it should ignore cost-worthiness judgments (at which point some services deemed necessary will be unaffordable, requiring another panel to determine affordability). Calling it a panel determining medical necessity is obfuscatory.

Hadorn (1992a) denies that the panel will make cost-worthiness judgments. Indeed, in his work with the state of Oregon, which I discuss in chapter 6, he suggests that we do not have to make such judgments because we can afford to offer everyone those medical services that are proved to bring necessary benefits. Hadorn helped Oregon revise its rationing list after it decided to abandon CEA. In place of CEA, Hadorn suggested that the state group health care services into seventeen broad categories, with life-saving services at the top of the list (regardless of their cost) and preventive services such as colon cancer screening lower down.

Hadorn's view that the cost of health care services can be ignored is naïve. It is naïve to think that we can easily afford to offer every proved beneficial health care service to every patient who would benefit from it. For example, we have solid evidence that colon cancer screening saves lives (Eddy et al. 1987; Mandel et al. 1993). Yet most experts recommend that screening should begin at age fifty. They make this recommendation not because screening would be useless in younger patients, but because colon cancer is extremely rare in people younger than fifty and, thus the cost of preventing death from the disease is extremely high. Recent diagnoses of advanced colon cancer in two prominent American baseball players, both under the age of fifty, show the consequences of this type of decision.

Whereas it may be appropriate to screen for colon cancer beginning only at age fifty, we should not kid ourselves that this decision is either a value-neutral "scientific" decision, or that it hinges somehow on the distinction between necessary and beneficial health care services. Unless Hadorn has a very strict idea of what it means to prove that colon cancer screening saves lives, or unless he would say that saving lives through screening is simply unnecessary in people less than fifty years of age, plenty of proved medical interventions such as these are available that we simply cannot afford to offer to everyone who would benefit from them. For this reason, it is important to separate discussions about whether specific health care benefits are necessary from discussion about whether they are affordable. By equating the withholding of necessary services with rationing, Hadorn and Brook make it too easy for others to ignore the difficult moral judgments crucial to any determination of necessary benefits.

Of course, it is possible to define rationing as withholding necessary services without relying on a panel of experts to determine what services are necessary. Hence, problems raised by Hadorn's reliance on experts do not necessarily doom his definition. Nevertheless, his definition has other problems. Most important, when we talk about necessary health care services, we have to ask, necessary for whom?, for what? Necessity cannot be determined without reference to some goal or external justification. If a fashion model wants a perfect face, cosmetic surgery may be necessary. But that does not mean cosmetic surgery should be included among necessary health care services. It is unlikely that a panel of experts would consider cosmetic surgery to be necessary. However, without such a panel, or some acceptable definition of necessary, we cannot determine whether withholding cosmetic surgery from fashion models is an example of rationing.

The word beneficial is also relative, and we can ask, beneficial for whom or for what? But the phrase beneficial health care service does not have the strong implications that necessary health care service does for resource allocation decisions. Necessary services seem, almost by definition, to be . . . necessary! We *must* provide them. Beneficial services, on the other hand, do not have to be provided. In fact, most people are probably willing to admit that cosmetic surgery is beneficial for fashion models while not wanting to make it part of any basic benefits package. (Of course, there is room to debate whether that type of cosmetic surgery constitutes health care.)

Determining which health care services are beneficial also requires difficult value judgments. For example, how do we decide when an unproved but theoretically promising treatment is beneficial? Nevertheless, determinations of which services are beneficial are less value laden than are determinations of which services are necessary, because they do not involve cost-worthiness judgments. If colon radiographs bring more medical benefit than flexible sigmoidoscopies, they are beneficial regardless of their financial cost. Expert panels deciding which necessary services to include in a basic benefits package must decide whether the additional costs of the film are justified. In contrast, panels deciding whether the intervention is beneficial do not have to make such cost-worthiness judgments. For this reason, some believe that decisions about determining basic benefits packages should not be made by expert panels, but instead by more representative bodies (Goold 1998).

A great advantage of defining rationing as the withholding of beneficial services is that it points out that it is no longer possible, if it ever was, to offer people every potentially beneficial medical service. Instead, determinations of which services are beneficial often identify those that are unaffordable. Difficult judgments about whether to offer them will no longer be made to look like scientific judgments about whether they are truly necessary. Instead, people will recognize the need to make value judgments about whether specific beneficial services can be offered to everyone.

In addition, we can use the negative connotations of beneficial to draw attention to difficult moral decisions about which services are worth pursuing. By focusing attention on our inability to offer beneficial services to all who need them, we can highlight morally questionable policies that create inequitable access to beneficial health care. It is not difficult to convince the public that allowing millions of people to be uninsured or underinsured is an example of health care rationing; yet, according to Hadorn and Brook's definition, this is not obvious. After all, laws in the United States require hospitals to provide emergency treatment regardless of patients' ability to pay. Lacking an agreed-upon list of necessary services, these laws could be interpreted as a guarantee that patients will receive necessary care. Consequently, if rationing is equated with the withholding of necessary services, uninsured people may be thought of as receiving necessary care, and the huge problem of having so many uninsured and underinsured people will no longer appear to qualify as rationing.

People do not like rationing. They should not like a health care system that allows so many people to go without adequate insurance. Equating rationing with withholding beneficial care highlights the terrible consequences of having so many uninsured and underinsured people.

Why I Prefer a Broad Definition of Health Care Rationing

I prefer a broad definition of health care rationing that includes any implicit or explicit mechanisms that allow people to go without beneficial services. By choosing this definition I am not suggesting that the term health care rationing has only one meaning. Instead, I am trying to clarify how I will use the term throughout the book. In addition, I hope this broad definition will be a useful starting point for debates about health care policy and health care priority setting.

I have primarily argued for this definition by pointing out problems with more restrictive definitions that seek to limit rationing to explicit mechanisms, absolutely scarce resources, or necessary health care services.

But another type of argument leads me to the same definition. As mentioned above, the dividing lines between absolutely scarce and non-scarce resources, between explicitly and implicitly withheld resources, and between necessary and beneficial resources, are not sharp. Take the line between beneficial and necessary health care services. Perhaps a more accurate representation of these distinctions would look like figure 2.8.

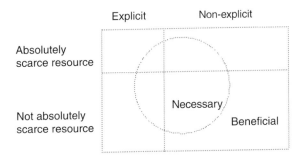

Figure 2.8
The fuzzy world of health care rationing.

Given their fuzziness, it seems arbitrary to limit rationing to any of the narrow definitions that rely on maintaining them. Instead, choosing a broad definition acknowledges their arbitrariness and focuses our attention more on whether particular health care services are appropriate to withhold. Although we could debate whether cosmetic surgery is necessary or beneficial, it is much more important to decide whether all patients who want a specific type of cosmetic surgery should receive it.

My definition of rationing encompasses many rationing decisions that do not strike most people as morally problematic and others that strike most people as unacceptable. It forces people to deal with the gray areas in moral debates about what patients ought to receive and what they should be allowed to go without. It forces us to deal with the moral issues in their full and troubling complexity.

By choosing this definition I have created room for many types of rationing, a number of which are suggested by the distinctions discussed above. There is explicit and implicit rationing, rationing of absolute scarce resources and of fiscally scarce resources, and rationing of necessary and of beneficial but unnecessary resources. Similarly, there are more and less justifiable types of rationing. In this broad definition rationing is not defined as de facto inappropriate. Indeed, a major advantage is that it forces us to decide when it is acceptable to allow particular patients to go without beneficial health care services.

This definition is not without problems. No consensus exists, for example, about what constitutes beneficial health care. As discussed above, some of this debate occurs because many health care services have not been studied enough to show whether they are beneficial. Other parts of this debate occur because of more unresolvable controversies. What should we do, for example, about therapies that are beneficial for some subgroups of patients but, when applied in aggregate, are not beneficial? I deal with some of these issues later in the book.

For now it is important to recognize that, amid great controversy about whether we should ever ration health care, the issue may have less to do with what services people think everyone should get than with how they define rationing. At a minimum, given tremendous variation in what people mean, those discussing it should state at the outset their definition. I have explained why I prefer a broad definition whereby rationing involves anything that allows patients to go without beneficial medical services. This view, combined with the negative connotations of the term, emphasizes the ubiquity of tragic choices in health care and highlights our need to decide what types of medical care we want everyone to receive.

I struggle every day with decisions about how far to pursue my patients' best medical interests in a climate of cost containment. Clinicians such as I could financially bankrupt the VA system where we practice if we ignored the costs of the diagnostic and treatment modalities at our fingertips. For us, health care rationing as I define it is a daily reality. But should it be? Is it right for anyone to withhold services from patients who could benefit from them?

3

The Necessity of Rationing Health Care

Imagine you and five friends have just finished stuffing yourselves at a fancy restaurant. The waiter rolls by with a cart filled with sumptuous artery-hardening desserts: chocolate mousse, baked Alaska (at least it's not fried!), and some kind of pie cowering below six inches of meringue. Despite having stuffed yourself, you have room in your spare "dessert stomach," and begin pondering your choices. Your waiter introduces each dessert with a pile of adjectives and . . . a six-dollar price tag!

You are crushed—your dessert stomach is simply not large enough to get six dollars of pleasure out of any of these offerings. Then, in a flash of inspiration, you remember that you and your companions are keeping only one check for the meal, meaning the cost of your dessert will be split six ways. You are confident in your ability to get a dollar's worth of pleasure out of one of these desserts. You order the chocolate mousse and prepare to nibble at its margins, confident that it will be a dollar well spent. Unfortunately, your five dinner companions, reasoning the same way you do (your friends aren't idiots!), also order desserts. As a result, each of you ends up paying full price for a dessert that none of you would have spent six dollars on.

Health care insurance, like a single check in a restaurant, distributes expenses across many people, creating an incentive to buy health care services that cost more than they are worth, a phenomenon health economists refer to as moral hazard (Fuchs 1996; Pauly 1968; Phelps 1992). Patients respond to health insurance the same way restaurant customers respond to shared checks: they purchase more goods (Keeler et al. 1988).

Because of insurance, people often spend more money on health care than they want to. They desire a routine blood test with very little chance of benefiting them because insurance picks up most of the cost. An expensive procedure that yields small benefits compared with an inexpensive procedure is preferred by physicians, who stand to do well by doing good, and by patients, who, more often than not, do not know the relative costs and benefits of the two. Physicians and patients do not care whether a CEA shows that the expensive procedure costs $200,000 per QALY. They only care that it is better than the less expensive one. In fact, for most people, the cost of health care and of health insurance is a mystery. Governments and employers pick up much of the cost of health insurance and deduct it from workers' salaries without their knowing its actual cost. It is almost as if health care consumers are not only splitting the check at a fancy restaurant, but are also turning the check over to their employers for reimbursement.

Health insurance increases demand for health care services, thereby promoting inflation. Fancy restaurants have little incentive to lower the price of desserts when customers split their checks and turn their receipts over to their employers (who, of course, receive a tax deduction for the expense). Similarly, health care institutions throughout much of the developed world have little incentive to lower their prices. Insurance decreases incentives for patients and clinicians to talk to each other about the costs of services, once again promoting inflation. And insurance creates high profit margins for medical technology companies, thereby encouraging the development of newer, more expensive technologies, thereby (you guessed it) promoting inflation.

To some, the ever rising costs of providing new, beneficial technology to patients leads to the unavoidable conclusion that health care rationing is both necessary and inevitable. Daniel Callahan, cofounder of the Hastings Center, an influential bioethics think tank, maintains that health care needs are limitless. Recent decades have seen great improvements in care and in health in most industrialized countries. Yet, the demand for further improvements continues to increase (Callahan 1987, 1990). Some experts point out that the costs are driven by a technological imperative (Churchill 1987; Eddy 1994; Emanuel 1991). Perhaps the only people who demand more insistently on an increasing number of high-tech gadgets in health care than professionals are patients. Combine this limitless need and ceaseless demand with an aging population, and we have a recipe for bankruptcy.

Others counter that rationing is neither necessary nor inevitable. Some say that it is unnecessary because health care is special, therefore, it is wrong to set any limits on health care goods (Lee & Jonsen 1974). Some believe that until we eliminate wasteful health care practices, it is premature to talk about rationing (Angell 1985). Others contend that, because the need to ration is caused by the inflationary effects of health insurance, we should simply eliminate or drastically reduce the amount of the insurance so that rationing decisions can be left in the hands of consumers.

When Oregon first unveiled its plan to ration Medicaid services, many questioned whether any state in the United States had to ration health care; with the federal government spending money on B1 bombers and with citizens spending money on sport utility vehicles (or whatever they were called back then), it made no sense for Oregon to do it. If these people are right, Oregon's cost-effectiveness list was doomed to fail no matter how it ranked health care services. Indeed, in a world without a need for health care rationing, CEA is irrelevant.

But CEA is not irrelevant. We do not live in a world where health care rationing is unnecessary. Although it is impossible to know what percentage of a country's gross domestic product (GDP) ought to go to health care, and impossible to prove that the United States, for example, is spending too much of its GDP on health care, I believe that many beneficial services that are routinely offered to patients are a poor way to spend money.

Why Health Care Rationing Is Necessary Even Though Health Care Is Special

Some people say rationing is unnecessary because health care is special. These people are half correct. Health care *is* special. Nevertheless, it still should be rationed.

Health care is special because life is sacred, and health care is one of the few goods and services that can prevent premature death. Steel-belted radial tires and a low home mortgage rate are not much good to a dead man.

Health care is also special because health is special. Good health is necessary before people can enjoy the most basic parts of life. A mountain bike does not bring much benefit to a person with crippling arthritis, and a good conversation is difficult to have during a migraine headache. Many things we value in life, and many goods and services we value in our economy, depend on people being healthy enough to enjoy them. More important, a certain level of health is necessary for people to have fair opportunities to pursue life goals (Daniels 1985). If we do not provide glasses for them, nearsighted children will be at a disadvantage in learning how to read and, therefore, in pursuing certain types of jobs when they are done with school. Untreated congestive heart failure makes almost any pursuit more difficult. Health care, of course, cannot provide equal opportunities or equal health for everybody. Some people are blind despite the best ophthalmologic care, and many people with congestive heart failure continue to have shortness of breath despite therapy. More-over, many factors influence health other than health care, including socioeconomic status, education, and genetics. But health care is one of the few commodities that can be vitally important to helping people achieve fair opportunity.

Because it is a special type of consumer good, people debate whether they have a right to health care. They are comfortable asserting, for example, that people have a right to basic nutrition if society can afford to give it to them. Like food, which makes life possible, health care, they insist, should be a basic right in advanced industrialized countries. Of course, health care is more expensive than food. But life is sacred, and thus we should not put dollar values on people's lives, nor should we worry about how much of our GDP we spend on health care.

But is health care so special that we should pursue its benefits at any cost? Is life so sacred that we should extend it regardless of the price?

An answer to these questions is suggested by the way we treat certain nonhealth care products that affect health. After all, health care services are not alone in their ability to improve health and prolong life. If we spent more money on road repairs, we could reduce traffic fatalities (table 3.1; Tengs et al. 1995). If we furnished every automobile-owning family

Table 3.1
Life-saving interventions and their cost-effectiveness

Intervention	Cost/Year of life
Mandatory automobile seat belt use	$69
Mammography for 50-year-old women	$810
Beta blockers for heart attack survivors	$850
Hypertension screening for men aged 45–54	$5,200
Grooved highway pavement	$29,000
Collapsible automobile steering columns	$67,000
Hypertension screening for asymptomatic women aged 20	$87,000
Colonoscopy for routine colon cancer screening	$90,000
Automobile air bags	$120,000
Breakaway rural highway utility poles	$150,000
Annual mammography for women aged 40–49	$190,000
Home smoke detector	$210,000
Adult monitors on school buses	$4,900,000
Six (versus 5) stool guaiacs for colon cancer screening	$26,000,000

Adapted from Tengs et al.

with a new Volvo, we might have a similar effect. If we established stricter environmental laws, we could probably reduce cancer deaths more effectively than by waiting until it is time for chemotherapy. Yet, we are willing, as a society, to debate how much money to spend on road repairs, automobile safety laws, and environmental protection. We ought to be equally willing to debate how much to spend on health care to promote these same ends.

Why are we willing to debate the cost-worthiness of solutions to some problems but not of health care? In part, because road improvements, automobile air bags, and environmental laws improve the health of unidentifiable "statistical" people, whereas many health care interventions are targeted at specific, identifiably ill people. A fifty-year-old woman needs emergency surgery: who is going to ask how much it will cost? But an engineer develops an expensive way to reduce traffic accidents and everyone wants to know how much it will cost and how many accidents it will prevent. Rightly or wrongly, people place significantly more value on saving identifiable lives than statistical ones (Jenni & Loewenstein, 1997; Schelling 1968). Since many health care interventions, especially the ones we see on television, are directed toward identifiably ill people, we mistakenly conclude that the cost of such life-saving services is irrelevant.

But of course, not all health care interventions save lives. Moreover, even some that are do not save identifiable lives but statistical lives. Blood pressure treatment reduces heart attacks and strokes. But not every patient with high blood pressure will have a heart attack or a stroke if untreated. Blood pressure control, like cholesterol reduction, Pap smears, mammograms, and exercise, helps unidentifiable, statistical lives. Similarly, new monitoring machines reduce the (already small) chance that patients undergoing surgery will have anesthesia-related complications. Hospital infection-control practices reduce the likelihood of hospital-acquired infections. But we cannot prevent all heart attacks, strokes, anesthesia complications, or hospital-acquired infections. Therefore, we should debate how much money to spend to reduce any or all of these events, and whether this money could be better spent elsewhere.

Whereas some health care services are special because of their ability to affect our longevity and our ability to pursue important goals, not all of them are special in this way. Instead, many of them offer small improvements in people's quality of life in ways that make it hard to distinguish them from a whole lot of other goods and services. Low back pain is one of the most common medical problems I encounter in my general medical practice (not to mention in my own life, which of course I have just mentioned). But relief of mild low back pain hardly rates as a service so special the we should not consider its cost. And many consumer goods and services improve quality of life more than relief of mild or moderate low back pain. I would have gladly put up with a month of low back pain for front row seats to see Michael Jordan play in a Bulls playoff game.

In fact, low back pain may be relieved as well by traditional nonhealth care consumer goods, such as well-designed office furniture and firm mattresses, as it is by health care interventions. Yet, health insurance pays for visits to physical therapists (sometimes) and for prescriptions for nonsteroidal antiinflammatory pain medications, but it rarely pays for mattresses or office chairs. Although insurance companies have to draw lines somewhere to limit expenditures for low back pain, health care is far from unique in addressing these kinds of problems. And outside of the health care market, money matters! Most of us are quite comfortable discussing how much money we are willing to spend on a mattress that might reduce our low back pain. We should be equally willing to discuss how much of our health care dollars we would spend to meet the same goal.

In summary, some health care services are special in the sense that it is unacceptable to even talk about cost-effectiveness when faced with an identifiable person in urgent need of them. But many services are not special in this way, and we ought to have an honest discussion about how much we should spend providing them.

Why Waste Elimination and Price Reduction Will Not Eliminate the Need to Ration Health Care

Some hold that health care rationing is unnecessary because costs can be adequately contained by eliminating waste (Brook & Lohr 1986). Experts estimate that roughly one-third of health care spending in the United States goes toward wasteful and unproved services (Brook & Lohr 1986). Numerous studies demonstrate substantial geographic variation in the use of expensive procedures that do not lead to measurable differences in health outcomes. A woman's likelihood of having a hysterectomy, an elderly man's chance of prostate surgery, and a child's chance of undergoing tonsillectomy all depend in part on where these individuals live (McPherson et al. 1982; Wennberg et al. 1988). If areas performing greater amounts of surgery are not achieving greater amounts of health, we should be able to save some money by reducing unnecessary surgery.

For those who think that rationing is unnecessary, it can further be argued that health care waste can be reduced by charging less for services. Do colonoscopies have to be as expensive as they are, for example? In a colonoscopic examination, a physician inserts a fiberoptic tube into a patient's colon to look for abnormalities. The examination is proved to reduce the chance that someone will die of colon cancer, because during the procedure polyps can be removed before they become lethal (Mandel et al. 1993). But colonoscopy often costs more than $500, causing some to accuse subspecialist gastroenterologists of "scoping for dollars."

Clearly, a great deal of wasteful medical expense could be eliminated by reducing the number of unnecessary procedures or by reducing their unnecessarily high costs. But even after all this waste had been eliminated, most industrialized countries would still be spending large portions of their GDP on health care, and the rate of increase in that spending would still outpace inflation (Emanuel 1991). Because health care is a very labor intensive industry, it does not experience the type of productivity gains that could reduce the cost of its services. Unlike computer hardware, for example, which grows more powerful and less expensive every year, health care services become more powerful and *more* expensive. Many new health care technologies result from increasingly complex research and development techniques. Gene therapy and artificial hearts promise to improve many lives, but they will not be priced to compete with a laptop computer any time soon.

The ability of waste elimination to reduce the need to ration health care is limited for another reason: waste elimination itself costs money. No magic wand can be waved that will make everyone stop wasteful health care practices. Instead, research to identify waste is expensive and is not easily translated into cost savings. Identifying waste is difficult because many interventions cannot easily be categorized as effective or ineffective. Instead, they are beneficial for some patients and not for others. It is a major challenge to figure out who will benefit from what. And, once we have this information, we must create mechanisms that will direct resources to appropriate patients. This, too, costs money, and at some point it may cost more to make sure that patients receive only beneficial care than it would to let some patients receive wasteful care.

Waste elimination even faces political obstacles. When the United States government created the Agency for Health Care Policy and Research (AHCPR), legislators hoped that the agency would help determine the most cost-effective way to spend health care dollars. The agency almost immediately ran into political nightmares. In reviewing data about low back surgery, for example, it concluded that many of these surgeries were wasteful and unnecessary. In response, a group of spine surgeons got together and almost succeeded in eliminating the agency (Deyo et al. 1997). The AHCPR has been almost incapable of funding new outcome studies for several years. Now cost-effectiveness analyses are more likely to be funded by industry than by this impartial agency.

Even if we successfully eliminate wasteful practices, some countries, especially the United States, would still face a major obstacle to containing costs—providing health care insurance for currently uninsured or underinsured people. To make sure everyone has a decent minimum of health care insurance would involve an increase in health care spending. It is unlikely that waste elimination would overcome this increase. (It is more than a little ironic that people in this country, in which 40 million are without health insurance, seem to be more opposed to health care rationing than people anywhere else in the developed world.)

Waste elimination also has a limited ability to eliminate rationing because many beneficial services are available that even the best-insured patients are currently not receiving. Take ambulances, for example. Rapid arrival of an ambulance can be life saving; but people living in rural areas are often far away from an ambulance, much less a tertiary care hospital. Thus, their emergency care services are compromised. If improving beneficial health care regardless of cost were really the goal, even after we had eliminated wasteful, nonbeneficial services, we would have to decide when to stop building ambulances. Similarly, consider the wonderful array of hospital beds available to reduce the chance that patients will develop decubitus ulcers. Some of these beds are enormously expensive, involving intricate channels of flowing air and sand that gently massage people's bodies and improve blood supply to their skin. These beds can be very helpful in preventing ulcer formation. (Of course, so can increasing the number of nurses per patient.) In any case, if no benefit is too small, we should spend the millions (and millions) of dollars it takes to equip nursing homes and hospitals with more of these beds. But we don't. At some point, society decided that the cost of an extra ambulance, or of an extra ulcer-preventing bed, is simply too much to pay for the small chance that it will help someone.

So far, I have tried to show why waste elimination is not a panacea for rising health care costs. But perhaps I should not be so worried about rising costs. If medical researchers come up with a cure for degenerative arthritis or congestive heart failure, won't those of us who suffer from these conditions be glad to shift more of our wealth into health care? What wouldn't most patients with Parkinson's disease pay to be cured?

It is crucial, however, to distinguish between debates about how much money we can or should spend on health care from those about whether we need to ration health care. Currently, approximately 15% of the U.S. GDP is spent on health care. Suppose we decided that we could afford to spend 25% in this way. That would mean that, if worthwhile medical therapies were available that were not being offered, we could spend money on them. Or, if new therapies were developed that were worth while, such as cures for degenerative arthritis, congestive heart failure, or Parkinson's disease, we could afford to pay for them. But it would not mean that we *ought* to spend 25% of our GDP on health care. We would still have to examine whether those services are worth while or, instead, whether some of the money spent on health care goods would be better spent elsewhere.

An early CEA showed that an inexpensive screening test for colon cancer, if repeated for a sixth time in a patient whose first five tests were normal, continued to find colon cancers, but at a cost of $26 million for every year of life gained. Debates about how much of our GDP we should spend on health care are irrelevant in light of this cost. However much we spend or however much we could ultimately afford to spend on health care, we should *not* spend money this way. Even if this screening test had no harmful consequences, most people would have to agree that $26 million is an awfully high price to spend for a year of life. Those who think it is not too high have only to think about the cost of repeating the test a seventh time—it would probably take more than $100 million to save a year of life. Thus CEA teaches us that after we spend money to achieve important benefits, further benefits often come at greater and greater financial cost. At some point, we must decide to stop pursuing these incremental benefits. At some point, we must decide to ration health care.

How Can We Reduce the Economic Impact of Moral Hazard?

In the opening of this chapter I explained that health insurance is a major catalyst for excessive spending because of moral hazard—the effect of sharing health care expenses through insurance on people's willingness to pay for additional services. Some may wonder whether we can avoid excessive spending, and maybe even rationing, by eliminating or reducing the economic impact of moral hazard.

Eliminating Moral Hazard by Eliminating Health Insurance

Any good waiter knows that the best way to increase how much food people order at a restaurant is to have them share their expenses on a single check. Any frugal restaurant patron (present company included) knows that the best way to reduce dining expenses is to keep separate tabs so you don't have to pay for your friend's third glass of scotch. We could similarly reduce health care expenses by eliminating health insurance, thereby requiring people (above some minimum income perhaps) to pay for their own care without anyone else's financial assistance.

In this way, patients' health care purchases would no longer be subject to moral hazard. Eliminating insurance would make patients less likely to request marginally beneficial care. It would also encourage them to examine the cost and quality of care. In theory, this would benefit patients by providing them only with services they deemed worth it. If a service is too expensive, patients will spend their money on more beneficial goods, whether they be other health care services or wall-to-wall carpeting. Eliminating health insurance would relieve society of difficult rationing decisions, because informed patients would decide whether the costs (monetary and otherwise) and benefits of their treatment options are worth while.

To be clear: eliminating health insurance would reduce health care expenditures, but it would not avoid health care rationing. Instead, it would ration according to willingness and ability to pay.

Of course, although eliminating insurance would lower costs and eliminate moral hazard, almost no one wants to eliminate insurance completely. Ability and willingness to pay are unacceptable bases for rationing many health care services. Often, these goods are not discretionary, yet purchasing them would be financially catastrophic to anyone other than Bill Gates. Some life-saving interventions, such as long stays in intensive care units, can cost hundreds of thousands of dollars, and many relatively common interventions cost more money than a typical person has available. Insurance smooths out predictable expenses, such as childbearing and prostate surgery, and distributes the expenses of unpredictable, highly expensive treatments among many people. Moreover, the mere thought of distributing some services by ability to pay is morally bankrupt. Who would ask a man with an acutely fatal condition whether he had enough money to save his life? Who would withhold a liver transplant from a dying woman simply because she did not have $400,000 in spare change? Because it is important to protect people from the often catastrophic expense of treating serious illness, we accept the economic inefficiencies of health insurance. If we want to control costs and reduce the economic impact of moral hazard, we should not do so by totally eliminating insurance.

Reducing Moral Hazard by Eliminating Health Insurance for Discretionary Services

Although it would be wrong to eliminate health insurance for all medical services, perhaps we could offer it for necessary services but eliminate it for unnecessary, or discretionary, services—the "dessert" of health care, if you will. Many health care goods are like an expensive dessert: they bring benefits, but the benefits are often not worth their financial cost.

Obstacles limit the role that out-of-pocket costs can play in the delivery of discretionary services. As discussed in chapter 2, it is extremely difficult to define necessary and beneficial medical care, much less to distinguish between them. It is similarly difficult to distinguish discretionary from nondiscretionary care. Even many chronic conditions, such as diabetes and emphysema, force people to spend large sums of money to avoid serious consequences. Are insulin syringes discretionary for a patient with adult-onset diabetes? How about glucometers? Are inhalers discretionary for patients with emphysema? How about home oxygen? Without an acceptable definition, or even a list, of discretionary services, using out of pocket costs to limit them is of minimal utility.

Some have thought that insurance copayment schemes are useful ways to separate necessary and discretionary services, by encouraging patients to decide what they need versus what they can do without. If patients have to pay even a portion of their health care bills out of pocket they will think twice about making unnecessary emergency room trips. Results from the Rand health insurance study suggest, however, that patients with copayments do not selectively reduce their use of unnecessary services (Brook et al. 1983). This was a randomized trial of health insurance coverage that, among other things, looked at the effect that different levels of copayment had on health care use and outcomes. The study showed that copayments caused a large decrease in expenditures with minimal impact on patient outcomes, raising hopes that asking patients to bear part of their health care costs directed them away from unnecessary services. However, further analysis of the Rand data showed that copaying patients were as likely to avoid necessary as unnecessary care; the financial incentive did not cause them to learn what care was necessary and what was discretionary (Lohr et al. 1986). This result raises questions about whether patients will have enough information to make optimal choices about what care they need and what is discretionary.

Requiring patients to pay out of pocket for discretionary services, especially marginally beneficial ones, is appealing. We already ask people to pay for smoke detectors, antilock brakes, fireproof children's clothing, and massage therapists, all of which probably improve health. Why not ask them to pay for expensive colon cancer screening tests, for better antinausea drugs, and for nonsedating antihistamines?

Industrialized countries, especially the United States, have to do a much better job of defining those services everyone should have access to versus those they must pay for versus those that should be unavailable to everyone. This is a very challenging task. It requires societies to define a decent minimum of health care and to make sure that this decent minimum is not eroded by allowing the middle and upper classes to purchase services it does not include. Health insurance is an important social good because it allows people to plan their lives knowing that they will not be financially crippled by the cost of receiving care for unforeseen illnesses. And many services are special goods that should not be denied simply because people do not have enough money. But health insurance, through moral hazard, drives up health care costs beyond what people would be willing to pay, and not all of the services are so special that money should be irrelevant. Therefore, society must find a way, other than by forcing people to pay out of pocket, to ration health care services.

Reducing Moral Hazard at the Time of Health Insurance Enrollment

Another way some propose to reduce moral hazard is to ask people to act like rational consumers at the time they purchase health care insurance (Menzel 1990). Rather than eliminating insurance or insurance for discretionary services, this proposal asks people to choose insurance plans according to services that are covered.

Imagine a healthy person deciding between two plans. The plans are identical except that one (slightly more expensive) promises to pay for lung transplants and the other does not. The person choosing can decide how much money she is willing to pay to be assured that lung transplantation will be available if she develops lung failure. In theory, if she has information about her chances of developing lung failure in the next year and the benefits and risks of various treatments (including lung transplantation), she should be able to make a rational choice between these plans. Consequently, she will end up with a plan that reflects how she would elect to spend her dollars.

Although this proposal is appealing, it has several problems. First, it creates the opportunity for adverse selection of patients. Adverse selection occurs when patients preferentially enroll in insurance plans that cover services that they need (Buchanan & Cretin 1986; Jackson-Beeck & Kleinman 1983; Robinson, Gardner, & Luft 1993). In the example above, the prices of the two competing plans are partly based on estimates about how many people are likely to require lung transplants. But if people who predict that they will have to have a transplant preferentially enroll in the plan that covers the procedure, that insurance company will have more transplant patients than it is prepared for. Any time insurance plans distinguish themselves by the services they cover, or the copayments they have, an opportunity exists for adverse selection.

Second, this model requires patients to learn and process large amounts of information. Insurers would have to be clear and specific about what services they provide, and people would have to grasp what these differences mean to them. Many people probably do not know enough about positron emission tomographic (PET) scans, for example, to know whether they want them included in coverage. It would be staggeringly difficult to decide whether to purchase insurance that covers prostate-specific antigen (PSA) blood tests, lung transplants, PET scans for brain disease, PET scans for other diseases, or myriad other options. Even if insurance companies could be convinced to describe their benefits in sufficient detail to allow comparison, potential enrollees would be overwhelmed, they would be unlikely to comprehend the information, thus, making informed choice impossible (Hibbard et al. 1998).

Third, for decisions on insurance enrollment to decrease health care costs, society would have to make people stick with their choices, even if that meant they would suffer. This could be heart wrenching, especially if, as in the example of lung transplantation, some insurance companies lowered their rates by eliminating expensive life-saving treatments. Many times, people are not good at predicting their future preferences (Kahneman & Snell 1990; Redelmeier, Rozin, & Kahneman 1993b). For example, patients may say they never want to go on dialysis, but when the time comes change their minds and give dialysis a try. This would put us in a position of either watching some patients suffer simply because they wrongly predicted their future preferences, or providing them care that they did not pay for, thereby undermining the whole idea of having them decide what services they want covered at the time of insurance enrollment.

Of course, it would be less heart wrenching to deny people services when those services do not involve life-saving interventions or interventions with huge impacts on quality of life. If someone chose an insurance plan that limited physical therapy appointments to two for treatment of chronic low back pain, or that paid for five well-baby check-ups in the first year of life rather than six, few of our hearts would be wrenched if those people later decided that they would have liked to have additional physical therapy or pediatric appointments. This suggests that asking people to make rationing decisions at the time they enroll in insurance plans might be more feasible if we allowed insurance companies to distinguish themselves only by which discretionary services they offered. This alternative brings us back to our discussion involving the challenge of defining discretionary versus nondiscretionary services while maintaining a decent minimum health care standard for all. This approach has great potential, but clearly a lot of work remains to be done.

A fourth challenge to having people decide on coverage at the time of enrollment is that most insurance or managed care plans do not differ by which services they explicitly cover. Instead, they differ by how aggressively the third-party payers contain health care costs. Although they may have explicit policies about the coverage of rare, expensive procedures, such as bone marrow transplantation for breast cancer, most of the difference in cost and quality is due to the aggressiveness of their utilization review process, to how efficiently they discharge patients from the hospital after surgery, and to how effectively they negotiate reimbursement rates with physicians and hospitals. These differences may affect quality, but not in ways anyone has yet been able to measure successfully. Consumers trying to choose plans that reflect their values will have a hard time determining these sometimes subtle, often immeasurable, differences.

CEA's Role in the Necessary Job of Rationing Health Care

Oregon's rationing decisions in the case of Coby Howard are impossible to defend. But in its later movement toward CEA, the state seemed to be heading in the right direction. Surely, some of its Medicaid dollars must have been going toward medical services that were not worth the cost. Certainly, CEA should have been able to help it identify such services.

Although CEA seems like an ideal way to identify health care services to ration, Oregon's experience convinced many people that the analysis will never be up to the task. Many people are convinced that it simply fails to capture public rationing preferences.

I will ultimately propose that CEA can help us identify which health care services to ration despite its inability to capture all the values important to our rationing decisions. But first, I want to take a look at people's values to see what it means to say that CEA does not perfectly capture public preferences.

4

The Challenge of Measuring Community Values in Ways Appropriate for Making Rationing Decisions

Imagine you have severe degenerative arthritis. Every trip up a flight of stairs sends sharp pains ricocheting from joint to joint. Short walks seem like long ones. Long walks seem like ancient history. To make matters worse, the pain pills you take give you stomach ulcers. On a scale from zero to 100, where zero represents health conditions as bad as death and 100 represents perfect health, what number do you think would capture your qualify of life if you had this type of severe degenerative arthritis?

An awfully difficult question to answer, isn't it! Coming up with a meaningful answer is a challenge. But without answers to questions like these, CEA would be unable to compare the benefits of arthritis treatments with the benefits of other treatments. Ultimately, when patients, physicians, health insurance companies, or governments make health care rationing decisions, they must make judgments about the relative importance of curing arthritis versus relieving symptoms of congestive heart failure versus about a billion other benefits.

Oregon's cost-effectiveness list did not fail because the people were opposed to health care rationing. This raises the possibility that the list failed because of cost-effectiveness—because CEA is not up to the task of demonstrating how society ought to set health care priorities.

But how do people want to set these priorities? How do health planners, cost-effectiveness gurus, and others figure out how people want to ration health care?

As challenging as it is for most people to provide a meaningful answer to the zero to 100 arthritis question, research and policy planners have an equally difficult time coming up with better methods of measuring people's rationing preferences. A look at several methods of measuring community values will show how challenging it is. Different methods yield different results, and no single method will ever perfectly capture people's preferences. But the process yields important information about what people want out of health care. As I will show in this and subsequent chapters, it tells us a lot about whether, or to what extent, CEA captures public rationing preferences.

Why Is It so Difficult to Measure Community Values in Ways Appropriate for Setting Health Care Priorities?

Facts alone will not show us how to set health care priorities. Even armed with complete knowledge about the cost and benefits of interventions, we must still combine these facts with public values.

It is difficult to measure these values. To begin with, no single community makes up our society, or any society (Emanuel 1991). Would the Roman Catholic community, for example, feel the same way about the importance of fertility services as other people? Could we even talk about *the* Roman Catholic community, when Roman Catholics themselves are parts of so many other communities and come from such disparate backgrounds? The first task here is to decide which community it is whose values we want to incorporate into health care policy.

It is also difficult to measure community rationing preferences because, once we have identified the appropriate community whose values to measure, such as enrollees in a specific health care plan or adult citizens of a state determining its reimbursement policies, we are left with the problem of how to find its values. The problem has two seemingly simply solutions. We could rely on consumer choices (for purchasing specific services or for purchasing health insurance), or we could rely on political processes to reveal community values. But unfortunately these seemingly simply solutions are insufficient.

As discussed in chapter 3, we cannot rely solely on the free market to reveal community values for how to ration health care. It is often inappropriate to sell health care through the free market—no one would want a poor person to die because she could not afford a life-saving appendectomy. Consequently, most interventions will be paid for, at least in part, by health insurance. Since insurance generates excess demand for services, the buying and selling of health care goods in a market dominated by insurance will not reveal the true value people place on those goods. Even for highly informed patients, we should not assume that their demands for services reflect their values; when part of the expense is picked up by insurance, their demands will potentially conflict with how they really would choose to spend their money.

Similarly, we cannot rely on people's choice of insurance plans to reveal their rationing preferences. Health insurers and managed care organizations rarely provide adequate information about the services they cover; and even if they did, people could not process it well enough for their insurance plan to capture all their values. Instead, their insurance enrollment decisions would, at most, be based on a limited range of values, such as whether a plan included their favorite physician or hospital, and whether it had good prescription coverage. Other values would be downplayed, leaving insurance companies and managed care organizations with difficult decisions about whether to pay for lung-reduction surgery, yearly Pap smears, smoking-cessation classes, or acupuncture therapy. Enrollment decisions simply cannot reveal community preferences for all of these different services.

We would similarly be mistaken to rely on political processes. Legislators require more community input about how people want to set health care priorities than they can glean from reading constituents' letters or from studying election returns. Health insurance companies and managed care organizations also must have more information about community values than can be determined from political mechanisms. Suppose a managed care organization is deciding whether to cover lung-reduction surgery to treat emphysema, an experimental operation that removes damaged tissue so that healthier tissue has more room to expand. Should members of the community sit in on the discussion to decide about this treatment? Would these individuals have to demonstrate their ability to interpret the scientific evidence for and against this surgery? Or would they sit, like a jury, listening to evidence presented by experts, and make a decision? Would enrollees be given the information and decide by vote whether to cover the surgery? Suppose we came up with an appropriate mechanism to decide about coverage for this controversial intervention. What about the hundreds and thousands of other coverage decisions insurance companies must make? Should the public be involved in formulary committee decisions? Or in the development of screening recommendations?

I would like to see many more governments and health care organizations experiment with ways of involving the community in coverage decisions. But ultimately, feasibility dictates that many, if not most, coverage decisions will be made without significant direct input from the community.

Because governments and insurers, who often play a large role in determining which services will be available, cannot rely solely on voting booths or free markets to tell them what patients want, they must have some other way to find out. They need some measure of community values.

The need for community value measures brings a third challenge to the surface. Most people in most communities have not spent much time thinking about health care priorities. Thus, community value measurement is as likely to reflect subtle aspects of the technique itself as it is to reflect people's deeply held beliefs about how to ration health care (Fischhoff, 1991).

With this challenge in mind, I review five common methods of measuring community values, and demonstrate how challenging it can be to make these measurements in ways useful for setting health care priorities. In subsequent chapters, I search for truth amidst the morass of data on the subject. Although we are far from discovering complete truth in these matters, and indeed are far from agreeing about whether there are any true measures of community values, I contend that we know enough about these values to improve the way in which they are incorporated into CEA.

Five Common Methods of Measuring Community Values

1. Quantifying community values in CEA measurement using utility assessment

Oregon's zero to 100 questions are an example of utility assessment. Cost-effectiveness analysis uses utility assessment to measure community values for the relative importance of various health improvements. For example, a health care intervention that improves a person from a condition worth a utility of 10 (on a scale from zero to 100) to a condition with a utility of 30 is said to bring the same benefit as an intervention that improves a person from 70 to 90, and to bring twice as much benefit as an intervention that improves a person from 70 to 80.

The actual numbers produced in utility measurement are unimportant. What is important is that the numbers place health conditions on an interval scale. It would make no difference if Oregon had used a scale ranging from 100 to 200. In fact, most utility measurements are converted to a scale of zero to 1 so that the maximum utility (of perfect health) is given a value of 1. Consequently, a year of perfect health is worth 1 QALY. Oregon's scale can easily be converted to zero to 1 by dividing people's responses by 100. A health condition with a utility of 50 on the scale of zero to 100 would have a utility of 0.5 when converted to a scale of zero to 1.

Strictly speaking, utility assessment does not measure *community* values, but *individual* values. Each individual person says what he or she thinks it would be like to live with a specific health condition. Nevertheless, these individual values can be aggregated to provide overall measures of how a community values various states of health. If a community of three people thinks that below-the-knee amputation has a utility of 0.2, 0.5, and 0.8 respectively, it has an average utility of 0.5.

Averaging utilities is morally questionable. Much like the election of a president who represents no one's first choice for the job, any aggregation of individual values into a community value measurement may end up truly capturing no one's values. On the other hand, there are few alternatives to such aggregation. Ultimately, if we are going to be making decisions for groups of patients, we may have to ignore individual variation in order to serve the interests of the larger group.

Beyond irresolvable controversies about whether it is appropriate to aggregate community values, utility measurement is controversial because no general agreement exists about how to best measure people's health care utilities (Richardson 1994). Many experts do not consider the rating scale used by Oregon to be a true utility measure because it may not place health conditions on an interval scale. Instead, they prefer standard gamble and time trade-off measures, which some think do.

In the standard gamble method of utility measurement, people are asked what chance of death they would take to rid themselves of a health condition (Froberg & Kane 1989). If they are not willing to take any chance of death, the condition is said to have the same utility as perfect health. If they are willing to risk a 40% chance of death, the condition is said to have a utility of 0.6 on a scale ranging from zero to 1, the most common utility scale in the CEA literature.

In the time trade-off method people are asked how many years of life they would give up to rid themselves of a health condition (Froberg & Kane 1989). Suppose a person can be expected to live fifty years with a disability. If he were just as happy to live forty years in perfect health as he would be to live fifty years with this disability, the disability has 4/5 the utility of perfect health, which translates to a utility of 0.8 on the zero-to-1 scale.

In addition to placing health states on an interval scale, the responses people give to standard gamble and time trade-off elicitations are thought to have inherent meaning, unlike their responses to rating scale elicitations. If people think seriously about what chance of death they would take to rid themselves of a condition, that number *means* something. A 10% chance of death is not an arbitrary number; it is a real risk that people have to think about. In contrast, the number 90 has very little intrinsic meaning.

Oregon's use of the rating scale to estimate the utility of health conditions rather than the standard gamble or time trade-off raises a question: would the cost-effectiveness list have captured public values more accurately if Oregon had used standard gamble or time trade-off measures? Were unacceptable rankings, such as placing more importance on TMJ splints than on life-saving appendectomies, a result of the rating scale? Or would standard gamble and time trade-off measures have created the same types of seemingly inappropriate rankings?

Do Utility Measures Predict Rationing Choices?

To see whether the failure of Oregon's list resulted from its use of the rating scale, several colleagues and I conducted a study to see how well utility assessment methods capture people's rationing preferences (Ubel et al. 1996c). On day 1 we elicited health-related utilities from a group of people for three conditions: mild hand pain, moderate knee pain, and severe, unrelenting headache pain. People were randomly divided into three groups based on the type of utility elicitation they received. One group received rating scale utility elicitations for each of the three conditions. These people read descriptions of the three health states and rated them on the zero to 100 scale. Another group received standard gamble elicitations and were asked to state the highest chance of death they would be willing to take to rid themselves of each condition. The third group received time trade-off elicitations.

Two weeks later, on day 2, we asked the same people to make rationing choices to see if their utility responses predicted their rationing choices. For example, suppose someone responded on day 1 that knee pain had a utility of 0.75. For his rationing choice to be consistent with this utility response, he should be indifferent between saving ten people's lives who could be returned to perfect health (thereby producing 10 QALYs per year), and curing forty people of the knee condition (improving them from 0.75 to 1.0, thereby producing, once again, 10 QALYs per year). We individualized the questionnaire so that all people received rationing choices for which they would be indifferent about which group to treat, *if* the choices were consistent with their utility responses. A person who thought the knee condition had a utility of 0.5 would be asked to choose between saving ten people's lives or curing twenty people of the knee condition. In contrast, a person who thought the knee condition had a utility of 0.9 would be asked to choose between saving 10 people's lives or curing 100 people of the condition.

What did we find? On day 1, most people rated the hand condition as being less severe than the knee condition, which was viewed as being less severe than the headache condition (table 4.1). In addition, each method produced the same ordering of health states; however, the

Table 4.1
Mean utilities for the health states as measured by the three utility-elicitation methods from day 1

| | Mean utilities* | | |
Health condition	Rating scale	Standard gamble	Time trade-off
Mild hand pain	0.92	0.91	0.99
Moderate knee pain	0.63	0.83	0.94
Severe headache pain	0.37	0.75	0.90

* On a scale ranging from 0.0, for conditions as bad as death, to 1.0, for perfect health.

utilities estimated by these different methods were quite different. The rating scale produced lower utilities than did the standard gamble and time trade-off methods, findings that are consistent with other research (Hornberger, Redelmeier, & Petersen 1992; Read et al. 1984; Torrance 1976).

What about people's rationing choices? We found that most people preferred treating the patients with the more severe condition significantly more than would have been predicted from their utility responses. The utility measures did not come close to predicting people's rationing choices, often off by factors of 100, 1,000, or more (table 4.2). In an extreme example of the discrepancy, the mean time trade-off utility for the hand condition on day 1 was 0.99, suggesting that saving 10 people's lives brings the same number of QALYs as curing 1,000 people of the hand condition. But when given a rationing choice, most time trade-off respondents felt that an infinite number of people would have to be cured of the hand condition to equal the benefit of saving ten people's lives.

Our study revealed, first, that the discrepancy between utility elicitations and rationing choices existed not only for the rating scale method used by Oregon, but was also true for the time trade-off and standard gamble elicitations. Thus, the failure of Oregon's CEA list cannot be blamed on its use of the rating scale rather than the other two methods. Second, the discrepancy existed not only when compar-

Table 4.2
Discrepancies between indifference points of rationing choices from day 2 and indifference points predicted by utility responses from day 1

Rationing example†	Median discrepancy between rationing choices and utility responses*		
	Rating scale	Standard gamble	Time trade-off
Appendicitis vs. headache	8.3	100.0	81.5
Appendicitis vs. knee	35.7	10,000.0	720.9
Appendicitis vs. hand	100.0	600,000,000	∞
Meningioma vs. hand	10.0	1270.0	100.0
Knee vs. hand	10.0	40.0	5.0
Meningioma vs. knee	44.3	3.3	10.0

* A discrepancy value of 100 means that the person's indifference point in the rationing survey was 100 times greater than that predicted by the utility response. For example, if the utility response indicated that he should be indifferent between curing 10 people of appendicitis and 100 people of headache pain, a discrepancy of 100 means that the actual rationing choice indicated he was indifferent only when $100 \times 100 = 10,000$ people would be cured of headache pain.
† Appendicitis versus headache refers to a paired choice between curing ten people of life-threatening appendicitis versus curing some number of people of headache pain, where the number is individualized for each respondent so it brings the same number of QALYs brought by curing appendicitis.

ing life-saving with nonlife-saving treatments, but also when comparing two nonlife-saving treatments, such as the headache condition and the knee condition.

The failure of Oregon's CEA list could have occurred in part because people's goal for spending limited funds is not solely to maximize health-related utility. In fact, wherever policy makers tried to set health care priorities according to CEA (not only in Oregon, but also in The Netherlands and New Zealand), it was abandoned as the basis of the priority system (Maynard & Bloor 1995). By relying on utility measurement to capture community values, CEA operates on the assumption that the goal of health care should be to maximize average health-related utility. But before accepting this assumption, we should find out whether the public agrees that health care money ought to be spent in ways that maximize health-related utility. In short, we must explore other methods of measuring community values to see whether people think the goal of health care ought to be to maximize measurable outcomes and, if not, to see what other values they think deserve a role in setting health care priorities.

2. Ranking the importance of specific health care services or distribution principles

Rather than rely on utility measurement to capture community rationing preferences, some researchers provide a list of health care services, or a list of categories of services, or a list of rationing criteria, and ask people to rank them from most important to least important (Bowling 1996; Jacobson & Bowling 1995; Klevit et al. 1991; Kliger 1995; Society of Critical Care Medicine Ethics Committee 1994). In this way, researchers can determine whether people want to ration health care solely in ways that maximize health outcomes or health-related utility or whether they value other goals, too.

Several researchers devised a list of sixteen health services and asked a group of British citizens to rank their importance (Bowling 1996). The citizens ranked treatment of children with life-threatening conditions as the most important priority, followed by care for dying patients; last on the list was cosmetic surgery. In a methodologically similar study, researchers asked a group of critical care professionals to review a specified list of priority-setting criteria and indicate which ones they thought were important in deciding which patients should be given the last available bed in an intensive care unit (Society of Critical Care Medicine Ethics Committee 1994). Most respondents indicated that the probability of patient survival was very important, whereas few thought a financial cost-benefit analysis was important.

Instead of providing respondents with a preestablished priority list to rank, researchers can have them create their own list and rank it. For instance, after abandoning CEA as the basis of its rationing plan, the Oregon Health Services Commission decided to elicit community values through a series of meetings in which they asked citizens to say what health care services or goals they believed were most important (Klevit et al. 1991). The discussions were open ended and the moderators, presumably, left it up to participants to generate a list. On reviewing the lists, the moderators looked to see which priorities were mentioned as being important at the greatest number of meetings. Oregonians (or at least those interested enough to show up at the meetings) said they valued disease prevention and quality of life at most meetings and cost-effectiveness at fewer meetings.

As opposed to utility assessment and CEA, the ranking approaches taken by these researchers do not assume that people think the goal of health care policies should be to maximize health-related utility. Instead, they attempt to find out what values people think should underlie their health care system. Indeed, several of these studies seem to indicate that cost-effectiveness is not viewed favorably by many. In the Oregon and critical care studies, for example, it was not ranked highly.

Nevertheless, we must be cautious about how we interpret studies asking people to rank short lists of health service categories or priority-setting principles. First, the categories or principles used in these studies are often not unique or discreet. In the survey of critical care professionals, for example, although cost-effectiveness was ranked near the bottom of the list, the four most highly ranked criteria were quality of life, probability of survival, reversibility of the disorder, and nature of the disorder. All four are crucial determinants of the cost-effectiveness of providing intensive care to any patient. Thus, the low ranking that critical care physicians gave to cost-effectiveness may not reflect rejection of CEA as much as it reflects that most of the important aspects of CEA were captured in other categories.

Second, asking people to rank principles or criteria is an abstract exercise. How should we interpret rankings of health care distribution principles when people do not have concrete examples of what these principles mean or of how the rankings will influence health care delivery?

Third, this approach involves aggregation of people's individual values into some type of group ranking. This is not surprising, since most measures of community values rely on some form of aggregation. Utility measurement, as we have seen, mathematically averages people's individual values. Ranking exercises, on the other hand, aggregate values in a way more similar to voting booths—researchers tally up votes for specific principles or criteria and see which ones come out on top. But, unlike utility measurement, they do not allow much opportunity to weigh the strengths of people's preferences. A person who thinks the top five rationing principles he ranked are almost equally important might not be distinguishable from another person who thinks the top three principles he ranks are significantly more important than the fourth and fifth principles.

Fourth, asking people to rank a small number of principles or criteria leaves us with an imprecise measure of values. For example, does the low priority given to cosmetic surgery in the British study reflect people's views of the importance of breast reconstruction after mastectomy or facial reconstruction after serious trauma? Can people's values be adequately captured by a list of sixteen health care services? Similarly, when people rank services without regard to the probability that they will produce benefits, it is unclear whether they truly think the service ought to be given priority. What does it mean to say that preventive services are more important than care of the dying? Does that mean that all preventive services are more important? What about preventive services that prevent disease in only a small percentage of people who receive them?

3. Rating the importance of specific health care services

One reason researchers usually provide only a short, and therefore imprecise, list of rationing criteria is because it is difficult for people to rank order large lists; consider the effort it would take to rank the importance of 200 health care services or 150 rationing criteria. In contrast, it is relatively easy to state one's opinion on each item in a long list by rating each service on a preference scale. Thus, an alternative to asking people to *rank* a short list is to provide them with a longer list and have them *rate* the importance of each item.

Fowler et al. (1994) gave an example of how this method can be used and why it avoids some of the shortcomings of ranking methods. They presented members of the general public with a sample of 227 clinical vignettes, such as the following:

A 40-year-old woman has had a cough for one week and now a temperature of 102° F and chills. The woman goes to see a doctor for examination and medication.

If you were designing a health insurance plan, what priority on a scale of 1 to 10 would you give this service?

People gave the highest priority to helping accident victims, patients with cleft lips, suicidal patients, and those who contracted the human immunodeficiency virus from a blood transfusion. They gave lowest priority to cosmetic surgery, treatment of scraped knee, and fertility treatments.

This approach is less blunt than the ranking exercises described in the previous section, in part because it provides people with a large number of cases to rate and thus gives a more detailed account of what services people value. Rather than ask people what importance they place on mental health services, Fowler et al. wrote vignettes of suicidal patients, severely depressed patients, and patients with marital problems who needed counseling. This approach is also less abstract than ranking exercises because it gives specific clinical examples rather than broad categories such as preventive care.

Although rating tasks can be more detailed and less abstract than ranking tasks, it is still often difficult to interpret importance ratings. How much more important, for example, should a priority score of 8 be than a priority score of 5? Unlike utility elicitations, where numerical values are placed on interval scales such that a change of two units is twice as large as a change of one unit, rating scales do not necessarily have interval properties. (Because the rating scale used by Oregon did not necessarily place health conditions on an interval scale, it probably deserves to be included with Fowler's rating study rather than with utility measures like the standard gamble and time trade-off.)

In summary, rating tasks provide more information about the strength of people's preferences than ranking tasks, but less information than utility elicitations. For example, consider the benefits of two treatments: cure of plantar warts versus cure of life-threatening appendicitis. It is easy to rank the benefits: treating appendicitis is more important than curing plantars warts. And, on a scale from 1 (for least amount of benefit) to 10 (for most benefit), it is easy to rate the relative benefits; most people would give them a 1 and a 10, respectively. But it is very difficult to say how much more benefit is brought by saving a life than by curing a plantar wart. Certainly, it is more than 10 times greater benefit. But, is it 1,000 times greater? 100,000?

4. Assessing people's willingness to pay for health services

Some researchers measured values for various health care services by asking people how much they would be willing to pay to receive them. One group of researchers interviewed patients in Great Britain who were waiting for cataract surgery and asked them how much they would be willing to spend to shorten their waiting time.

Willingness-to-pay measures seem to hold great promise for measuring community values. Wouldn't it be useful for British legislators to know how much people would pay to shorten waiting time for cataract surgery? Wouldn't it be nice to know how much U.S. veterans would pay for Viagra versus how much they would pay for the PSA test to screen for prostate cancer? These methods are a very direct way of measuring the importance people place on specific health care services. They also have the advantage of being relatively comprehensible. People make willingness-to-pay decisions every day. This stands in sharp contrast to time trade-off utility elicitations, for example. People do not think very often about how much time living in perfect health would be equivalent to living the remainder of their lives in less than perfect health. These measurements share many of the advantages of rating exercises, too, in that people can be asked about their willingness to pay for many different health services and their responses can be used to rate the relative importance of these services. Moreover, these numbers have more meaning than most rating scale responses. Rating a health care service on a scale from 1 to 10 has less meaning than saying how many dollars one would be willing to pay for it.

But, at best, willingness-to-pay surveys provide a messy approximation of the value people place on specific health care services. First, although people are used to making such decisions in everyday life, they are not used to making them about most health care interventions, because they usually pay for these with health insurance. Thus, people have not been faced with the true dollar value of most of the health care goods they have received. This is not a fatal flaw in willingness-to-pay measurement, but it is one to be reckoned with. These measurements are best when they approximate the types of decisions people would make in everyday life.

Second, the estimates are often insensitive to the quantity of goods being bought. For example, studies estimated how much people are willing to pay to prevent 1,000 acres of land from being deforested. This figure is nearly identical to what they would pay to prevent 2,000 acres from being deforested (Baron 1996). A similar phenomenon could damage the validity of health care willingness-to-pay surveys. Imagine someone who says he would spend $1,000 to prevent himself from developing colon cancer. How much would he then spend to prevent himself from developing brain cancer? Thyroid cancer? Lung cancer? . . . The list goes on. And what about other types of diseases? At some point, this man would simply not have another $1,000 available to prevent some tragic illness. More important, he may not have been thinking about all the other types of cancers or illnesses he could develop when he said he would spend $1,000 to avoid colon cancer. In conducting willingness-to-pay surveys, researchers must focus respondents on the item being measured while reminding them of all the other things they might want to spend their money on.

Third, these measures are a bad way to estimate the value of life-saving services. How much would you spend to save yourself from immediate death? I would spend everything I had plus everything I could borrow. Does that mean the cost of life-saving medical services can never be too high?

In summary, willingness to pay is a promising way to measure community values, especially for nonlife-saving services. But this method

alone is not an adequate measure of community values. It must be supplemented by other techniques.

5. Experimental survey designs to reveal factors that subconsciously influence people's stated values

Utility, ranking, rating, and willingness-to-pay measures ask people
consciously to evaluate health care treatments or conditions. But people's values may be subconsciously influenced by factors that cannot
be discovered through these methods. For example, if asked whether it
is better for a treatment to have a 10% mortality rate or a 90% survival rate, most people would say that the two are identical. Yet, studies employing experimental survey designs showed that people place
different values on health care treatments when their effects on survival rates are described versus when their effects on mortality rates
are described (McNeil et al. 1982). Subtle differences in how information is framed can affect people's judgments.

In experimental surveys, descriptions of items being evaluated (be they
clinical situations, abstract categories of health services, or health care
rationing vignettes) are altered so that different respondents receive different descriptions. This alteration across questionnaires makes it possible to see how people's stated values are influenced by the
descriptions. My colleagues and I used an experimental survey to explore attitudes toward allocation of scarce transplantable kidneys
(Ubel et al. 1996b), a topic mired in controversy because of racial inequities in how kidneys are distributed in the United States. The current system places a heavy emphasis on antigen matching in
distributing available kidneys, because it slightly improves transplant
outcomes. This emphasis on antigen matching places African-Ameri-
can patients at a disadvantage because they have rarer antigens than
Caucasians. In the United States, African-Americans wait an average
of eighteen months for a transplant, compared with nine months for
Caucasians (Ayres, Dooley, & Gaston 1993; Gaston et al. 1993).

We wanted to see what the general public thinks of the trade-off between antigen matching and waiting time in kidney transplantation: is
it fair to let one group of patients wait twice as long as another because they have rare antigens simply to improve transplant outcomes

by 5% or 10%? At the same time, we were unsure about how to elicit these values. Asking people how the racial identification of patients with rare antigens ought to affect kidney allocation creates potential for biases consciously or subconsciously to influence their responses. If Caucasians stated that antigen matching ought to be given great emphasis regardless of which racial group suffers, how confident would we be that this emphasis was uninfluenced by their knowledge that matching favors Caucasians?

To overcome this problem, we varied the description of the kidney transplant system across several surveys. In one version we told subjects that antigen matching causes African-Americans to wait twice as long as Caucasians for transplants, and in another, that antigen matching causes Caucasians to wait twice as long. In yet another we eliminated all mention of race and said that antigen matching causes people with blood types B and O to wait twice as long for organs as people with blood types A and AB (Ubel et al. 1996b). (Blood type actually does predict waiting times and transplant outcomes for the same exact reason that race does; people with relatively rare blood types tend to have relatively rare antigens.)

We found that these different ways of presenting the information influenced how people chose to allocate scarce organs. Any mention of race, regardless of whether antigen matching favored whites or blacks, caused people to place less emphasis on antigen matching and thus less emphasis on maximizing transplant outcomes. In contrast, people receiving the blood type version, where race was not explicitly mentioned, were significantly more inclined to distribute organs on the basis of antigen matching to maximize outcomes, even though this created disparity in waiting time. It seems that the disparity in waiting time was not as worrisome when people were unaware that it caused racial inequities.

Experimental surveys are extremely helpful in determining how people respond to small wording changes. People may respond differently to a questionnaire about tuberculosis than they do to one about "consumption." Subtle and seemingly innocuous word changes, or even the order in which questions are asked, can influence responses. In a famous example of this, an annual survey of the U.S. population found one year that overall life satisfaction had significantly diminished from previous years, even though employment rates and other factors seemed unchanged. The pollsters finally realized that the life satisfaction question had been placed after a series of questions about recent deaths in the family, or some similar sorts of depressing questions. By the time people got to the life satisfaction part of the questionnaire, they had thought so much about who had died in their family that they reported that they were less satisfied with their lives. Thus surveys effectively help identify the influence of such factors.

Surveys are not only helpful in identifying subconscious factors influencing people's expressed values. They also indicate how people's expressed values change when specific factors are made explicit. In studying attitudes toward kidney allocation, we could have presented all three examples to the same subjects, asking them first to allocate organs according to blood type and then according to race. We could have even asked people to explain any differences in their allocation preferences across examples. This is not the place to go into great depth about the relative strengths of within-subject versus between-subject survey designs. Instead, I merely want to point out that these designs can be mixed and matched, thereby allowing researchers more flexibility in studying people's values.

A limitation of the designs, however, is that they do not necessarily show which surveys capture values the best. Does explicit mention of race make people's kidney transplant allocation preferences more or less valid? If patients with tuberculosis are viewed more favorably than those with consumption, which values should guide allocation decisions? In addition, surveys do not necessarily allow researchers to quantify the relative importance of various factors in influencing allocation choices, where one can say, for example, that X is twice as important as Y.

Community Values and CEA

As we have seen, CEA measures community values through utility assessment. The main advantage of utility assessment over many other measures is that it provides quantitative estimates of the relative importance people place on health changes brought by health care interventions. We can say that two QALYs are twice as valuable as one QALY. But we cannot say that a health care intervention with an importance score of 10 is twice as importance as one with a score of 5. The disadvantage of utility assessment is that it assumes that people's primary goal for spending scarce health care dollars is to maximize health-related utility. Perhaps people do not think that two QALYs for an elderly person are twice as important as one QALY for a child.

Some alternative methods discussed in this chapter suggest that people do not want to ration health care solely according to CEA. But the research presented so far is inconclusive. In the next chapter I present some more robust evidence exploring whether CEA captures people's rationing preferences.

5

How Do People Want to Ration Health Care? Balancing Cost-Effectiveness and Fairness

Imagine you are a famous transplant surgeon holding a heart in your hands. Its muscles quivering, you must transplant it as soon as possible. Two patients in the local hospital are deathly ill with congestive heart failure. Both are perfect matches for the heart. One patient is a sixty-year-old convicted murderer whose heart is failing because of a traumatic injury sustained when one of the thirteen children he massacred tried to defend himself. The other is a thirty-year-old Peace Corps volunteer who contracted heart failure from a virus common to the remote region of the underdeveloped nation where he was helping poor people. Both candidates have the exact same chance of benefiting from transplantation, including the same life expectancy, despite their difference in age. Both are likely to die within a week without a heart. Who would you choose to receive the heart?

If you are like most people, you would select the Peace Corps volunteer, a younger man who developed heart failure while trying to improve the world. But if you base your decision on CEA, you would be forced to flip a coin. Transplanting these two patients would be equally cost effective. Neither man would deserve priority over the other.

It seems that CEA ignores many important moral values when dealing with such situations. This moral emptiness is especially surprising, since CEA was picked as the economic measure of choice for health care because it was supposed to be morally superior to a more traditional economic measure, cost-benefit analysis, or CBA.

One way to understand the distinction between the two is to consider the distinction between medical utilitarianism and general utilitarianism.

Utilitarianism is a theory of distributive justice that holds that the best social policies are those that maximize overall happiness, or utility (Mill 1863). But CEA is distinct from utilitarianism in that it focuses only on health-related outcomes. It is better thought of as *medical utilitarianism,* the belief that health care dollars should be spent in ways that maximize measurable health outcomes. Medical utilitarianism is distinct from more general forms of utilitarianism because it focuses exclusively on measurable health outcomes, whereas general utilitarianism focuses on all outcomes. Medical utilitarianism values health care services solely according to their ability to improve people's health, whereas general utilitarianism also values how the services influences people's general happiness, whether health related or not. If an intervention improves a patient's health but decreases someone else's happiness, that is accounted for in general utilitarianism.

In CBA, which strives to account for the values of general utilitarianism, analysts measure the overall economic impact of health care interventions (Gramlich 1990). If an intervention improves the health of an elderly person who is no longer working and is drawing money from Social Security, this will be reflected in CBA. Prolonging the life of elderly people who are draining Social Security budgets is not very cost beneficial! In contrast, CEA measures health outcomes and says that health improvements in old fogies are worth just as much as similar improvements in young fogies. The fact that young people are more likely to be employed and old people are more likely to be receiving Social Security is irrelevant.

Cost-effectiveness analysis is the chosen form of economic measurement in health care because many people have moral objections to CBA. Cost-benefit analysis would place less value on treatments directed at elderly people and those directed at women, because both groups are less economically productive than young men. It would similarly discount the benefits of treatments aimed at people of low socioeconomic status.

Because CEA focuses so narrowly on health outcomes, it ignores other factors that potentially ought to play a role in health care allocation decisions. In the heart transplant dilemma, CEA would ignore the circumstances causing heart failure in these two very different patients and would also ignore their age differences. Do people think maximizing health outcomes should be the primary goal of health care spending, or do they think that other values ought to guide decision making?

In this chapter I present evidence about how people want to ration health care, and show that these preferences often conflict with CEA and its emphasis on health maximization. However, I also show that this seeming rejection of CEA is muddied by inconsistency and outright confusion among many about how health care ought to be rationed. This confusion is understandable given the complexity of most rationing dilemmas. Nevertheless, it also makes it more difficult to know what to do about people's rejection of CEA. Confused values do not easily translate into good health care policies.

Public confusion about how society ought to ration health care should not surprise us. Even many experts are confused. Who among us is without contradiction? Philosophers spend entire careers trying to develop logically consistent, plausible, and practical theories to guide policy decisions such as how to spend health care dollars. Even then, most of them end up contradicting themselves at one point or another, or leave some very important questions unanswered. So, even though the data I will present about public rationing preferences paint, at best, a fuzzy picture, this fuzzy picture will reveal some very plausible shortcomings of CEA that suggest directions in which it could be improved, and also explanations for why Oregon's list was rejected.

Public Preferences for Giving Priority to Severely Ill Patients, Even When Their Care Is Less Cost Effective

Suppose you were dictator for a day, a benevolent dictator, of course. And suppose you had a large sum of money to spend on one of two possible health care programs. The first program would bring moderate health benefits to 100 children stricken with a severe disease. The second would bring similar benefits to 100 children stricken with a less severe disease. Which would you choose?

Faced with this incredibly hypothetical dilemma, most people would chose to help the children with the severe disease from a feeling that, all else equal, scarce health care resources ought to go toward helping those in greatest need who have the most severe illnesses or disabilities.

In the previous chapter I discussed a study in which my colleagues and I found that people's responses to utility elicitations (e.g., zero to 100 rating scale) are not consistent with their rationing choices (Ubel et al. 1996c) For example, people who think that an injured knee has a utility of 0.8 on a scale from zero to 1 would still rather save ten people's lives, bringing ten QALYs per year, than cure fifty people of the knee condition, even though this also brings ten QALYs per year. When given a choice between helping two groups of patients who stand to gain equal QALYs, people almost always prefer to help those with the more severe illness.

Yet, CEA measurement is not concerned with how severely ill patients are who are receiving treatment, but with the number of QALYs brought by treatment (the average utility with treatment minus the average utility without treatment). Severity of illness is accounted for only in the way it influences the amount of treatment benefit. Slightly ill patients, for example, can at most receive slight benefits from treatment. Therefore, when severely ill patients receive only modest benefits, they receive the same priority as moderately ill patients who, for the same cost, receive the same benefits.

Some critics contend that CEA does not place enough priority on helping severely ill patients (Hadorn 1991; Jonsen 1986). The importance of helping the neediest is the basis of some important philosophical theories of justice (Miller 1976; Rawls 1971; Winslow 1982) and is present in many debates about the allocation of scarce medical resources (Barber 1987; Bryant 1973; Cohen 1996; Rawles 1989). It is even factored into transplant allocation, which gives priority to urgently ill candidates, even when their chance of benefiting from the procedure is less than that of other patients (Ubel, Arnold, & Caplan 1993; Ubel & Caplan 1998). It is also captured by some triage policies that give priority to helping the most severely ill patients (Baker & Strosberg 1992; Elster 1992).

In accordance with these philosophical arguments and policy positions, empirical evidence suggests that many people believe that severely ill patients deserve some priority in how we allocate scarce health care resources. Erik Nord, a Norwegian economist, conducted a series of studies on this issue. In one study, he presented members of the Norwegian general public with a policy dilemma involving how best to allocate

Project X	Project Y	Disability level
		1. No problems walking.
		2. Can move about without difficulty anywhere, but has difficulty walking more than a kilometer.
		3. Can move about without difficulty at home, but has difficulty up and down stairs and outdoors.
		4. Move about with difficulty at home. Needs assistance up and down stairs and outdoors.
		5. Can sit. Needs assistance to move about both at home and outdoors.
		6. To some degree bedridden. Can sit in a chair part of the day if helped up by others.
		7. Completely bedridden.

Figure 5.1
An example of two health care programs that improve disabilities by two levels, thereby producing the same number of QALYs. Which program would you choose?

funds to benefit people with various levels of disability (Nord 1993b). He described a hierarchy of seven disability levels (figure 5.1), selected because they were equidistant on a utility scale developed by Harry Sintonen. In other words, improvements in health from level 5 to level 3 bring the same number of QALYs as improvements from level 7 to 5.

In the policy dilemma, people were told that there was not enough money to treat patients with each level of disability and they had to decide whom to treat. Then they were given a series of choices in which patients differed in the initial severity of disability and in the amount of benefit they could obtain from treatment. The choice was between improving 100 patients from disability level 7 to level 5 and improving some other number of patients from level 5 to 3. People were asked how many patients had to be improved from level 5 to 3 so that they would have a hard time deciding which of these two groups of patients to treat. Nord varied the choices over a wide range of disabilities and found that people rarely specified numbers of patients in each treatment group that would bring equal QALYs. Instead, they placed additional importance on how severely ill patients were. Small improvements in severely ill patients were seen as being more important than larger improvements (in QALYs) for less severely disabled patients.

My colleagues and I repeated this study in the United States in a survey of people waiting to be assigned to jury duty at the Philadelphia County Courthouse, with one important twist: for half of the examples we asked people to choose among treatment programs that did not cure or improve disabilities, but instead that *prevented* patients from becoming more severely disabled (Ubel et al. 1998b). We wondered whether people still preferred helping more severely ill patients when considering the benefits of preventive interventions. In all honesty, I expected that respondents would prefer giving preventive services to the healthiest patients and curative interventions to the sickest. I thought they would think preventive care is most important in people who are already healthy. However, I was wrong. People preferred giving both preventive and curative interventions to the sickest, most disabled patients, even when the patients gained fewer QALYs than those who were less sick. A series of other studies show a similar pattern. People place more emphasis on treating severely ill patients than would be predicted from their utility elicitation responses (Nord 1991; Prades 1997; Ubel et al. 1998a).

Although suggestive, these results do not prove that people prefer helping severely ill patients over less severely ill ones. The discrepancy between utility measures and resource allocation decisions might have occurred because the utility measures failed to place health states on an interval scale. For example, improvements from disability level 7 to level 5 in Nord's study may have been larger than improvements from level 5 to 3.

To eliminate a faulty utility scale as an explanation for preferences for helping severely ill patients, Nord (1993b) presented people with the following example.

Imagine an illness A that gives severe health problems and an illness B that gives moderate problems. Treatment will help patients with illness A a little, while it will help patients with illness B considerably. The cost of treatment is the same in both cases. There is insufficient treatment capacity for both illnesses, and an increase in funding is suggested. Three different views are then conceivable.

1. Most of the increase should be allocated to treatment for illness B, since the effects of these are greater.
2. Most of the increase should be allocated to treatments for illness A, since these patients are more severely ill.
3. The increase should be divided evenly between the two groups.
Which of these views comes closest to your own?

Very few respondents favored allocating most of the increase to moderately ill patients, even though these patients would benefit more from treatment than severely ill patients. Instead, the largest number preferred dividing resources equally between the groups, and most of the remaining people favored treating the severely ill patients. This suggests that CEA's undervaluation of treating severely ill patients is the result of a fundamental clash between people's values—to treat severely ill patients first— versus the underlying values of CEA—to maximize measurable health benefits, or QALYs.

Nord's study is provocative, but his wording of the three conceivable views is flawed. For example, in his description of view 1, he did not remind respondents that illness B is only moderately severe, and in view 2 he did not remind them that patients with illness A benefit only a little from treatment. In addition, the wording of views 1 and 2 contain compound justifications. For example, in view 1, Nord provided an allocation preference, that "most of the increase should be allocated to treatment for illness B," and a reason for this preference, "since the effects of these are greater." Some people may prefer increasing the allocation to illness B for other reasons and would have difficulty choosing this view.

To follow up on and extend Nord's study, I presented his survey to prospective jurors in Philadelphia. But rather than sticking with the original wording, I randomized people to receive one of six questionnaires, only one of which (Q1) replicated Nord's original wording. In Q2, for example, I clarified the wording of the three views:

1. Most of the increase should be allocated to treatments for illness B, involving moderate health problems that improve considerably with treatment.
2. Most of the increase should be allocated to treatments for illness A, involving severe health problems which improve a little with treatment.
3. The increase should be divided evenly between the groups.

Because research shows that people make different allocation choices when considering their self-interests (Nord et al. 1993), in Q3 I asked people to think about their own self-interest when making a policy recommendation:

In making your policy recommendation, consider the possibility that you will be a patient affected by this policy and that you have an equal chance of developing either illness A or illness B.

Table 5.1
Treatment preferences for severely or moderately ill patients across three questionnaires

Questionnaire version	Description of questionnaire	N	People expressing preference for treating (%)		
			Illness A*	Illness B†	Equal for A & B
1	Original wording	76	26	9	64
2	Clarification	77	6	21	73
3	Self-interest	78	12	13	75

Not all percentages add to 100 due to rounding.
* Illness A: severely ill patients who improve slightly with treatment.
† Illness B: moderately ill patients who improve significantly with treatment.

In Q1, which replicated Nord's original wording, I confirmed his original results: 64% of respondents gave equal priority to these two groups, 26% favored treatment for severely ill patients, and only 9% favored treatment for moderately ill patients. But this pattern of responses was significantly altered in Q2 and Q3. Q2, which merely clarified the wording, revealed a significant decrease in the percentage of people who favored treatment for severely ill patients, although most still preferred giving equal priority to the two groups (table 5-1).

This preference for giving equal priority to the two groups raises the question of what group people would prefer if they were forced to make a choice. As I discuss later in this chapter, a common theme in surveys of public rationing preferences is that people do not want to make difficult choices. Thus, their preferences for equality in these hypothetical examples may reflect this unwillingness as much as it reflects a view that patients deserve equal treatment.

To see what people would do when forced to choose between treating severely or moderately ill patients, I randomized respondents to receive three other questionnaires. These questionnaires replicated the wording from Q1 through Q3, except they no longer gave people the explicit option of dividing the funding increase evenly between the groups of patients (view 3 from Q1 through Q3). In Q4, which replicated Nord's original wording, a slight majority preferred allocating funds to severely

Table 5.2
Responses to questionnaires where people were not given the explicit option of dividing resources equally between patients

Questionnaire version	Description of questionnaire	N	People expressing preference for treating (%)	
			Illness A*	Illness B†
4	Original wording	75	57	43
5	Clarification	78	40	60
6	Self-interest	77	42	57

Not all percentages add to 100 due to rounding.
* Illness A: severely ill patients who improve slightly with treatment.
† Ilness B: moderately ill patients who improve significantly with treatment.

ill patients, even though they benefited less from treatment. But in the two alternative wordings (Q5 and Q6), a slight majority preferred allocating funds to moderately ill patients. In none of these three questionnaires did preferences for moderately or severely ill patients reach statistical significance (table 5-2).

In summary, a number of studies suggest that people place special priority on helping severely ill patients ahead of others, even if their health care brings fewer QALYs. In fact, utility, and QALY, measurement undervalues the importance of helping severely ill patients. Thus, one problem with CEA may be that utility measurement, as it is currently done, does not place health states on an interval scale. However, Nord's study of Norwegian health care policy planners and my follow-up study suggest that utility measurement is not the main culprit here. Even in plain language, when we explained that severely ill patients would benefit less from treatment, many people wanted to give them priority or felt they deserve equal priority with less ill patients who would benefit more from treatment.

Many powerful criticisms of CEA seem to be explained by this preference for helping severely ill patients even when they gain fewer QALYs. When Oregon's CEA rationing plan was rejected for ranking TMJ splinting ahead of appendectomies, David Hadorn (1991) wrote that CEA violated the rule of rescue, a concept introduced earlier by Jonsen (1986), which holds that people want to help desperately ill patients ahead of others. Studies showing a discrepancy between utility elicitation and rationing preferences could be empirical evidence for a rule of rescue—people want to help severely ill patients even when that is not cost effective.

Public Preference to Avoid Discrimination Against People with Chronic Illness or Disability, Even When Their Treatments Are Not Cost Effective

Imagine two groups of patients stricken with a life-threatening illness. The first group was previously in full health and can be returned to full health with treatment. The second group previously had paraplegia and, with treatment of their life-threatening condition, will continue to have paraplegia. (For the purposes of discussion, assume that the utility of paraplegia is 0.8.) As shown in figure 5.2, in conventional CEA, saving the life of a person with paraplegia for a year produces 0.8 QALYs, whereas saving someone's life who can be returned to full health for a year produces 1 QALY. This suggests that saving the life of a person with paraplegia is only 80% as valuable as saving the life of someone who can be returned to full health.

The emphasis on maximizing QALYs in CEA conflicts with some people's attitudes toward the importance of saving the lives of patients with disabilities and chronic illnesses (Harris 1987; LaPuma & Lawlor 1990; Nord 1993a). In fact, quality of life measurement has come under significant criticism from people with disabilities for being discriminatory (Hadorn 1992b). Even Oregon's Medicaid plan ran into trouble for a while because its emphasis on quality of life measurement was believed to violate the Americans with Disabilities Act (Sullivan 1992). If the quality of life of people with disabilities is less than optimal, their lives will be given less value.

Early empirical evidence suggests that many people do not want to discriminate against patients for whom life-saving treatments will bring fewer QALYs because they have chronic illness or disability. Nord gave a group of Norwegians a choice between saving the life of a person who could be returned to full health with treatment versus saving the life of a person who could not be returned to perfect health but would live with

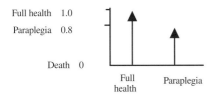

Figure 5.2
Two life-saving treatment programs: one saves the lives of patients who can be restored to full health and the other saves the lives of patients with preexisting paraplegia.

moderate disability (Nord, 1993a). Most respondents showed no preference for either patient but considered them equally deserving of intensive care treatment. Similarly, I gave prospective jurors a choice between saving the lives of 100 patients who could be returned to perfect health after treatment or some number of lives of patients with preexisting paraplegia. They had to say how many paraplegics' lives would have to be saved so that they would be unable to decide which group to save. Over 80% of people said that paraplegics' lives were just as valuable as others. In other words, saving the lives of 100 paraplegics was just as important to most people as saving 100 "normal" lives.

These two studies offer only limited proof that people think CEA undervalues life-saving treatments for patients with chronic illness or disability. Further research is necessary to see what value people place on treatments for patients with other disabilities. However, given intense criticism that CEA discriminates against people with disabilities and the potential that some CEA measures may place less value on the lives of these people (Harris 1987), it is plausible to think that further research will support the tentative conclusion that people reject QALY maximization when lives are at stake and some of those lives involve people with chronic illness or disability.

But is it fair to criticize CEA for discriminating against people with chronic disability or illness? After all, it is designed to evaluate programs and interventions at the population rather than the individual level, and it is rare that a given life-saving program or intervention is uniquely useful to a group of people who have a particular illness or disability (Russell et al. 1996). Analysts do not calculate the cost-effectiveness of coronary artery bypass surgery in subpopulations on the basis of paraplegic or nonparaplegic. They would have no plausible reason to separate out these groups on the basis of the effectiveness of the intervention. And no evidence in the literature indicates that analysts seek to discriminate explicitly against subgroups. However, in accounting for values, it is the exceptions that one must look to for instruction. It is important that CEA be able to account for a life-saving intervention that is specific to a particular illness (e.g., protease inhibitors for patients with AIDS) and, hence, to a particular group of individuals. Moreover, CEA experts have called on analysts to refine their analyses so that the calculation of treatment benefits takes account of patients' underlying health (Fryback & Lawrence 1997). A CEA of the treatment of life-threatening infections in persons with AIDS would have to account for their less than optimal quality of life after the infection is treated. A CEA of angina treatment would have to account for other chronic diseases affecting the typical patient with the disorder. In summary, most CEAs currently do not distinguish between whether or not health care interventions are specifically directed at people with chronic illness. As the measures become more refined, however, we will have to worry that life-saving interventions for people with chronic illness or disability will be given less value.

Public Preferences for Fair Distribution of Health Care Services or Health Care Outcomes

So far I have described two public values that currently are not incorporated into CEA. First, people want to give priority to severely ill patients, even if those patients do not gain as many QALYs from treatment. Second, they want to give equal priority for life-saving treatments to people with chronic illness or disability, even though by definition the patients will gain fewer QALYs from treatment. In both cases, it appears that people reject health maximization as the sole goal of health care spending.

Both values can be understood as examples of preferences for distributing health care services with attention to both efficiency and equity. Certainly CEA emphasizes efficiency—distributing health care services in ways that maximize health improvements. But people also want to emphasize equity or fairness in the most general sense of these terms. It does not seem fair to give lower priority to severely ill or disabled patients just because their health care is not as efficient.

In a series of studies, my colleagues and I explored attitudes toward the trade-off between equity and efficiency. As will be clear from reviewing these studies, people think the efficiency with which society distributes health care resources must be balanced with the perceived fairness, or equity, of this distribution.

Colon Cancer Screening: Efficiency or Equity?

Imagine the following:

The Federal government has set up a program to test for colon cancer in people enrolled in Medicaid, a government program that offers health insurance to low income people and families. The test allows doctors to find colon cancer at an early stage. So far, the government has offered the test to people at high risk of developing colon cancer, and has prevented many of them from dying of colon cancer. Now it wants to offer the test to the rest of the people receiving Medicaid, all of whom are at equally low risk of getting colon cancer.

A group of doctors was formed to help the government decide which of two tests to offer the low risk people. Test 1 is inexpensive but does not always detect cancers in their early stages. Test 2 is more expensive but is also better at detecting early cancers. The decision is complicated by budget limitations—the government only has a certain amount of money available to pay for the screening tests. After evaluating the costs and benefits of each test, the doctors reached the following conclusions:

The budget is just large enough to offer *Test 1* to all the low risk people. Under this program, *everyone can receive* the test. By doing this, *1000 people* will be prevented from dying of colon cancer. The budget is just large enough to offer *Test 2* to one half of the low risk people. Under this program, *half the people can receive* the test and half cannot receive the test. By doing this, *1100 people* will be prevented from dying of colon cancer.

To find out whether people want to maximize health outcomes, even if that means an unequal distribution of health care services across a population, my colleagues and I presented the example to members of the general public, members of a prominent bioethics organization, and members of the Society of Medical Decision Making, a group that has been instrumental in developing techniques for measuring the cost-effectiveness of health care services (Ubel et al. 1996a).

Unlike some of the severity studies discussed above, this example is unambiguous about which choice would maximize health. Test 2, the more expensive and more effective test, saves more lives than test 1. No matter how we measure health related utility, test 2 brings more health benefit.

We found that most of the general public and medical ethicists recommended offering test 1 to the entire Medicaid population, even though test 2 saves more lives (table 5.3). Nearly half of medical decision experts, many of whom conduct CEAs for a living, also recommend test 1. That result was especially surprising to me because, in CEA parlance, test 2 "dominates" test 1—it yields greater health benefits for the same amount of money. When one health care intervention dominates another, decision-making experts consider this to be a no-brainer; the dominated option should not be chosen. In fact, many computer programs designed to perform CEAs would eliminate test 1 from the final analysis because it is dominated by test 2. Nevertheless, these CEA experts showed that they are uncomfortable with the distributive implications of health maximization, when maximizing the number of lives saved requires an unequal distribution of health care resources.

How could people recommend test 1 over test 2 and allow 100 people to die whose lives could have been saved? Of the 388 people who recommended test 1, 305 justified this decision on the basis of fairness. For example, one person wrote, "It would be unfair to only offer the test to half the people." Another wrote, "Equity is more important than efficiency." And another, "It is not fair to randomly distribute health care." Eighteen people recommended test 1, not because they thought it was more fair, but because they were concerned about political appearances. One wrote, "Politics. Test 2 would be perceived as rationing, and thus unfair. People think in ways that are not always correct." Another wrote, "The indigent have been discriminated against for so long that a test that was available only to one-half of them would likely be viewed as unfair." And twelve recommended test 1 because the difference in survival between tests was too small to justify offering a test to only half the population. As one wrote, "The difference of 100 lives is not significant enough to use random selection."

Rightly or wrongly, many people thought fairness deserved enough role in making policy decisions that they would let 100 people die whose lives could have been saved. This is a response to a very specific example

Table 5.3
Colon cancer screening test recommendations

	% of respondents		
Recommendation	Prospective jurors (n = 568)	Medical ethicists (n = 74)	Decision-making experts (n = 73)
Test 1 (saves 1000 lives)	56	53	41
Test 2 (saves 1100 lives)	42	43	56
Refused to make a recommendation*	2	4	3

* These people provided written explanations for their refusal to make a policy recommendation.

involving Medicaid patients and a screening test for which it is hard to know who really benefits. How do people think about the trade-off between efficiency and equity in other circumstances?

Transplantation Allocation: More Evidence that the Public Values Fair Access to Health Care, even when It Diminishes Health Outcomes
Solid organ transplantations present an opportunity to study allocation dilemmas in which people have no choice but to agree that resources are limited. With respect to colon cancer screening, some people thought that the example was artificial and that the government should simply offer the better test to everyone rather than force people to choose between fairness and efficiency. For heart, liver, and kidney transplantation, however, there is no such option; not enough organs are available for the patients requiring them. Consequently, increasing numbers of people are on waiting lists. At the end of 1991, in the United States over 1,500 people were waiting for cadaver livers, and over 2,000 were waiting for cadaver hearts. By the end of 1997 these numbers had grown to 9,937 and 3,969, respectively (data from United Network for Organ Sharing). As the list grows, so too do the number of people who die before they can receive an organ.

Because of the unavoidable shortage of organs, the transplant community has literally had to decide, by choosing who gets an organ, who lives or dies. To those of us interested in the role of CEA in allocating scarce resources, this raises an obvious question: do people think that scarce transplantable organs ought to be allocated in ways that save the most lives? What other factors ought to be important in these allocation decisions?

My colleagues and I conducted a series of studies in which we described transplantation allocation dilemmas. The results confirmed the major finding of our colon cancer screening study: people do not always choose to allocate scarce health care resources in ways that maximize health benefits.

A Blood Test Predicting the Chance of Surviving Transplantation
Imagine the following:

Suppose that 200 children are waiting to receive a liver transplant, none of whom has any other health problems. They need to receive these transplants within one year or they will die. In that time, only 100 usable livers become available. Children who do not receive a transplant will die. A blood test is available that divides the children into two groups, each with a different chance of surviving transplant. No other information predicts their outcomes as reliably as this blood test.

George Loewenstein and I presented members of the general public with this example and randomized them to receive various information about the prognoses predicted by this blood test (Ubel & Loewenstein 1996b). In one questionnaire we said that the blood test divided the children into a group of 100 with an 80% chance of surviving if transplanted and 100 with a 70% chance of surviving. In other versions, the prognoses of the two groups of children were said to be 80% and 50%, 80% and 20%, 40% and 25%, and 40% and 10%.

If the sole goal of transplant allocation should be to maximize the number of lives saved, people should give all 100 organs to the children with the better prognoses. Yet, in all five questionnaire versions, most respondents did not allocate organs that way. In the 80/70 questionnaire, for example, only 13% gave all the organs to the group with the better prognosis. At most, in the 80/50 questionnaire, only 33% did so (table 5.4).

Rather than maximize survival rates, many people preferred to divide the organs equally between the groups. In the 80/70 version, most preferred equal allocation of organs, and in the 80/20 version, over one-

Table 5.4
Allocation decisions: Percent of organs allocated to the better prognostic group

Organs given to better prognostic group (%)	People making choice in each survey version (%)					
	80/70* (n = 32)	80/50 (n = 33)	80/20 (n = 34)	40/25 (n = 35)	40/10 (n = 35)	Total (N = 169)
<50	3	0	0	9	3	3
50	53	33	26	40	14	33
51–75	22	27	21	14	29	22
76–99	9	6	29	11	37	19
100	13	33	24	26	17	22

* E.g., 80/70 refers to the questionnaire version where the better prognostic group had an 80% chance of survival if transplanted and the worse prognostic group had a 70% chance.

fourth did. This last figure is notable because most transplant surgeons, an aggressive group if there ever was one, would probably not choose to transplant a patient who had only a 20% chance of surviving.

In many versions, large numbers of respondents chose to allocate organs in ways that struck a balance between equality of distribution, where each group of patients received half the organs, and efficiency of distribution, where the better prognostic group received them all. Overall, 41% chose to give somewhere between 50% and 100% of organs to patients with the better prognosis.

Of note, whereas fewer people would allocate organs in ways that maximized survival, most still preferred to give more organs to patients with better prognoses. In addition, as the difference in prognosis between the groups increased, so did the number of organs that people chose to allocate to patients with the better prognosis. When the prognostic difference was only 10% in the 80/70 version, more than half of the people would divide organs equally between the groups. But when there was a 60% difference in absolute survival in the 80/20 group, only one-fourth divided the organs evenly. In short, although maximizing lives saved is important, people do not think it should be the sole goal of transplant allocation. And, although distributing organs fairly is important, it should not be done without some regard to efficiency.

How do people justify allocation decisions that do not maximize the number of lives saved (Ubel & Loewenstein 1996a)? Eighty-one people wrote that patients *deserve a chance* of transplantation regardless of prognosis, writing, "Needy people deserve transplants, whatever their chance of survival," and "If I or my child were a member of either group, I would want a fair chance of receiving a transplant." Twenty-four respondents considered transplant *prognosis to be too unpredictable* to determine allocation, such as one who wrote, "Special circumstances in 50% group could enhance candidates' chances of survival." Ten people believed the prognostic information, but did not think that it warranted giving all the organs to group 1: "A 10% difference in survival does not seem significant enough to prompt more availability to transplants," and "I could justify giving the livers to children who had a 100% chance of survival and denying them to children who had a zero percent chance of survival. Any other ratio (90% vs 10%, 80% vs 20%, 70% vs 30%, etc. etc.) becomes increasingly difficult." Six people would give a small number of organs to patients with worse prognoses because they wanted research to be done to improve the chance that such patients would have a better chance of surviving in the future. One person wrote, "I believe in God. God doesn't work in numbers," and another, "*Do not* put any children through all the trauma and pain of surgery just on the pretense he/she *may* have a slight chance to survive!" Of interest, this last person gave 20% of the organs to a group of candidates with a 10% chance of survival, suggesting that by "slight chance" she meant something less than even 10%.

Many respondents used a combination of reasons to justify their allocation decisions. For example, one person receiving the 40/10 survey version gave 90% of the organs to the better prognostic group, stating, "I would like to save as many lives as possible and still give hope to the group that has the least chance to survive." A person receiving the 80/70 survey version gave 60% of the organs to the better prognostic group: "If the children in group 1 have a greater chance of survival, then the greater percentage of livers should be given to them. However, the children in group 2 should not be denied the chance for survival altogether just because that chance is more slim." These people, in effect, were trying to strike a balance between equity and efficiency.

Other Examples

Many people prefer an equitable distribution of transplant organs among groups of patients, even if that slightly decreases the benefits of transplant. For example, they want to give priority to patients awaiting a first transplant ahead of those needing a second or third transplant beyond any effect that retransplant has on outcomes (Ubel & Loewenstein 1995). Similarly, they give lower priority to cigarette smokers and intravenous drug users, even when these patients do better than others, and even when these patients' "socially undesirable behavior" is *not* responsible for their primary organ failure (Ubel, Baron, & Asch 1999). As discussed in the previous chapter, people's desires to maximize transplantation benefits are significantly diminished when they discover that a maximizing allocation scheme would disadvantage people of specific races (Ubel et al., 1996b).

The Message So Far: Rejection of CEA

The colon cancer screening and transplant studies suggest that many people do not want to allocate scarce health care resources in ways that maximize health benefits. When taken together with earlier studies showing that people want to give priority to severely ill patients and people with chronic disabilities even when those patients do not gain the same number of QALYs as others, results suggest that CEA promotes health maximization without adequate regard to issues of fairness or distributive justice. Health maximization is important to people, and so are issues of fairness that are not captured by CEA.

Okay, Fairness Is Important, But What Do People Mean by Fairness?

It is relatively simple to say that people think fairness ought to play an important role in health care allocation, but it is not so easy to determine what people mean by fairness. Imagine a painful condition that can be treated only by a scarce new drug. A physician has been give a daily supply of forty-eight pills to divide between two patients. For an hour of pain relief, one patient needs three pills and the other needs one. How should the physician distribute pills between these patients?

When this example was presented to a group of people, most gave thirty-six pills to the first patient and twelve to the second, thereby equalizing the amount of pain each patient experienced rather than the number of pills each patient received (Yaari & Bar-Hillel 1984). In a follow-up study, psychologists Kahneman and Varey (1991) told people to imagine that each patient initially required one pill for an hour of pain relief and that the physician gave each one twenty-four pills per day, thereby completely relieving both patients' pain. People were then asked to imagine that one of the patients became tolerant to the agent and now required three pills for an hour of relief (thereby mimicking the original problem posed by Yaari and Bar-Hillel). In contrast to Yaari and Bar-Hillel, they found that most people did *not* distribute pills in a way that equalized the amount of pain between patients. Nor did they continue to distribute pills equally. Instead, most gave somewhere between twenty-four and thirty-six pills to the patient who developed tolerance to the drug.

This shows that fair distribution schemes may differ from fair *redistribution* schemes. People do not want to take resources away once patients become used to receiving them, even if the final distribution is less fair or less efficacious. In the pain pill example, pain relief is not maximized, since the greatest relief would be gained by completely relieving pain in the nontolerant patient and giving the rest of the pills to the one developing tolerance. Nor is pill distribution equalized. Redistribution in this case encouraged people to compromise between equity and efficiency.

Fairness and equity are complex concepts, debated and refined by philosophers, theologians, and political theorists for thousands of years. It should not be surprising that subtle changes in allocation examples can have a large effect on what people perceive to be fair distribution. In a series of studies, my colleagues and I explored the consistency, or lack of it, of people's attitudes toward the role of fairness versus efficiency in the allocation of scarce resources. As with the pain pills, many of these studies show that people's preferences are greatly influenced by seemingly subtle, sometimes irrelevant, alterations in circumstances. Such inconsistency raises difficult questions about whether people's preferences are stable (and appropriately sensitive to subtle, but morally relevant differences) or whether they are a sloppy mess.

Is the Importance of Fairness "All or Nothing"?

Earlier I described a study in which my colleagues and I found that most people would rather offer a less effective cancer screening test to 100% of a Medicaid population (thereby saving 1,000 lives) than offer a more effective test to 50% of the population (thereby saving 1,100). What do people mean when they say they value fairness in such instances? Some might think the less effective test is more fair because it can be offered to *more people* than the more effective one. Others may think it is more fair because it can be offered to *everyone*. In other words, the value placed on fairness in this situation may depend on whether the more fair test can be offered to everyone.

To see whether preferences for fairness are all or nothing, a group of us conducted a follow-up study in which we randomized people to receive one of three questionnaires. In Q1 we replicated the previous study. In Q2 and Q3 we changed the percentage of Medicaid enrollees who could receive the two screening tests. In Q2, only 90% and 40%, respectively, of enrollees could receive the two tests, determined randomly by Social Security number. And in Q3, only 50% and 25%, respectively, could receive the two tests. In both Q2 and Q3, we told people that test 1 and test 2 saved 1,000 and 1,100 lives, respectively.

As with the previous study, most respondents receiving Q1 favored the less effective screening test that saved only 1,000 lives but could be offered to 100% of the population. However, in Q2 and Q3, only a minority of people favored the less effective test (table 5.5). This dramatic reduction in preference for the "fairer" test was seen not only in members of the general public, but also in a group of physicians. This result suggests that some people's preference for fairness over efficiency may be all or none: fairness loses value when a health care intervention cannot be offered to an entire population.

The dramatic reduction in preference for the fairer test in this study does not in itself suggest that preferences for fairness are fragile. After all, a test that cannot be offered to everyone must be distributed unequally, raising important moral concerns. Many people, in fact, wrote that they were disturbed by any random distribution of beneficial health care services. Some were concerned that the randomness would not be random. Others found randomness itself morally unacceptable or politically infeasible. Looked at another way, in Q1, people were asked to

Table 5.5
Colon cancer screening follow-up study: Percentage of people favoring the less effective screening test

Questionnaire version	Percent of Medicaid enrollees receiving:		Percent of people favoring Test 1, the less effective screening test	
	Test 1 *(saving 1,000 lives)*	Test 2 *(saving 1,100 lives)*	General public %(n)	Physicians %(n)
1	100	50	56 (166)	59 (434)
2	50	25	27 (169)	26 (423)
3	90	40	28 (160)	38 (437)

compare a fair test with an efficient one. In Q2 and Q3, they were asked to compare two unfair tests, thereby focusing on the greater efficacy of test 2.

Is the All or Nothing Preference for Fairness Arbitrary?

If the value people place on fairness depends on whether a health care intervention can be offered to an entire population, their preference for fairness over efficiency may depend simply on how a situation is described to them. After all, the definition of "an entire population" is often arbitrary (Baron 1995). Usually, we can find a broader population that includes the patients in question, which means some people are always excluded. What happens to preferences for fairness when we bring attention to this broader population?

In another follow-up to our colon cancer screening study, we randomly distributed five versions of a questionnaire to the general public. As in our two previous studies, we said that test 1, the less effective and less expensive test, saves 1,000 lives and that test 2, the more effective and more expensive test, saves 1,100. However, in this second study, we varied the proportion of Medicaid enrollees who could receive each of the two tests across two situations in each version. That is, people received two different examples. In the *all-tested* one, test 1 could be offered to 100% of Medicaid enrollees and test 2 to 50%. In the *half-tested* example, test 1 could be offered to 50% and test 2 to 25%.

We also varied the order in which people received the two examples. In Q1 and Q3, people first received the all-tested one. After making a recommendation, they were informed on the next page of the questionnaire that the Medicaid population had doubled and that the two tests could now be offered to only 50% and 25% of the population, respectively, saving the same number of lives.

In Q2 and Q4, people first made recommendations for which test to offer in the half-tested example. On the next page, we told them that the Medicaid population had decreased, because of a change in the Medicaid law, at which point they had to make a recommendation for the all-tested example. In Q5, people received both examples simultaneously on the first page of the questionnaire and were asked to make policy recommendations for them both on the second page. (By random assignment, the layout of Q5 was varied so that half the people received the all-tested example on the left-hand page and the other half received it on the right. We found no differences based on the page orientation.)

Finally, we varied whether enrollees in the first and second examples were from the same or different states. We hypothesized that once people had made a decision in the first example they would be reluctant to change their minds in the second, especially if the second involved the same group of enrollees [much like the reluctance to take pain pills away from patients demonstrated in the study by Kahnemann and Varey (1991)].

Table 5.6 shows our results. As we predicted from the results of our first follow-up study, preference for the less effective test was diminished in the half-tested example. However, the percentage of people favoring the less effective test also depended on the order in which they received the two examples and on whether the examples involved Medicaid enrollees from the same or different states. In Q1, 61% favored the less effective test in the all-tested example, consistent with our two previous studies; in contrast, in Q2 only 49% and in Q4 only 42% favored it. These differences can be explained in part by the order with which people received the examples. In Q1, the all-tested example was the first one people received. Their preference for the less effective and fairer test was predictable, given results of our two prior studies, when the all-tested example was the first (and only) one people received. But, in Q2 and Q4,

Table 5.6
Results of second colon cancer follow-up study: Highlighting the arbitrariness of screening an entire population

Questionnaire version	Order of the two examples	Whether the two examples involve the same or a different state	N	People favoring less effective test (%)	
				All-tested*	Half-tested†
1	All-tested first	Same	135	61	53
2	Half-tested first	Same	132	49	25
3	All-tested first	Different	107	50	49
4	Half-tested first	Different	121	42	25
5	Simultaneous	Different	120	42	32
Overall			615	47	32

* The two screening tests could be offered to 100% and 50% of the population, respectively.
† The two tests could be offered to 50% and 25% of the population, respectively.

people received the half-tested example first, and only 25% favored the less effective, fairer test. (This result, too, is consistent with our previous follow-up study.) But when Q2 and Q4 respondents then received the all-tested example they did not choose test 1 as often as those who received this example first, perhaps because they had already been primed by the half-tested example to favor efficiency over fairness. This priming was also prevalent in Q1, where most people still favored the less effective, but fairer, test in both the all-tested and half-tested examples, as if the former, which they received first, had primed them to favor fairness over efficiency.

These results seem to indicate that people's ideas of fairness and efficiency are, to put it bluntly, a mess. Put another way, their preference for fairness versus efficiency depends not only on how a situation is described, but also on which of two situations is described first. The importance people place on offering services to "an entire population" is arbitrary. If we call people's attention to the broader population, their judgments reverse. Indeed, in a separate study we described an option for a health maintenance organization (HMO) that operated in two states but could offer colon cancer screening in only one. The same people received narrow and broad descriptions of the test. In the narrow description, they were told what percentage of the population in state A would receive the tests. In the broad description, they were told what percentage of the HMO enrollees in both states received it. This is essentially a different way of describing the *exact same situation* because, in either description, people are aware that half of the HMO population lives in a state that won't receive colon cancer screening. Nevertheless, people responded differently depending on which description they received.

These studies suggest that people's preferences for fairness over efficiency when a health care service can be offered to an entire population are, in part, what psychologists call framing effects. They are significantly influenced by how the allocation example is framed, even when the difference between the framings is morally irrelevant. We should be cautious about interpreting preferences for fairness versus efficiency until such framing effects are more clearly understood.

When Is Fairness a Value and When Is It Innumeracy?

Another caution is in order when interpreting people's expressed preferences for fairness and efficiency: we must determine whether the preferences have been influenced by innumeracy. Earlier in this chapter I described a transplant prognosis study in which people were asked to distribute 100 transplantable organs among 200 children who were divided into prognostic groups on the basis of a blood test. To find out whether people understood, at the simplest level, the effect that their allocation decisions would have on aggregate survival, we asked the following question after they had made their choices: what distribution of organs to children in groups 1 and 2 do you think would save the largest number of lives? Most respondents did not realize that giving all the organs to the better prognostic group would maximize survival. Of special significance, a number of people responding to the 80/20 questionnaire not only distributed 80% of the organs to the group with an 80% chance of survival, but also believed that this distribution would maximize survival.

A number of studies show that people mistakenly think that they can maximize outcomes by "probability matching." For example, Gal and Baron (1996) gave people a series of dice rolls using a die with four green sides and two red sides. Each time people correctly predicted the color of a roll, they would receive a reward. Many people guessed green two out of three times, failing to understand that the optimal strategy would be to guess green every time.

We must be very cautious in interpreting people's responses to allocation examples to make sure we know to what extent their choices reveal their attitudes toward fairness versus their inability to grasp how to maximize outcomes.

When Is Fairness Unwillingness to Just Say No?

Another caution is in order when interpreting people's attitudes toward fairness. Sometimes allocation preferences may reflect inability to make difficult rationing decisions. People do not want to deny health care to groups of patients, yet, setting priorities often means making hard choices. When these choices involve denying health care to specific groups, many look for a way to avoid making the choices (Calabresi & Bobbit 1978). When people were asked to give priority to one of two patients requiring intensive care, only one of whom could gain full recovery from treatment, they did not want to deny treatment to the patient who had less chance of full recovery (Nord 1993a). Does this reflect the importance people place on equality in distributing scarce health care resources, or their reluctance to abandon a patient in need, even one who is less likely to benefit from treatment? My colleagues and I found similar reluctance to abandon patients in our transplant studies, in which many respondents, although they gave most organs to people with better prognoses, still gave a small number to those with worse prognoses (Ubel et al. 1996a, b, c; Ubel & Lowenstein 1995). How else can we explain why some people give ninety organs to patients with better prognoses and ten to those with worse prognoses? People simply cannot abandon a whole group of patients, leaving them without any hope.

In one study people were more willing to base allocation decisions on prognoses when patients were ranked as *individuals* compared with when they were divided into prognostic *groups* (Ubel & Lowenstein 1995). Imagine that 200 candidates can be ranked from 1 to 200 on the basis of their chance of surviving transplantation. People are relatively comfortable distributing organs to the top 100 patients, which excludes those with the worst prognoses from receiving organs. Yet, if the top 100 patients are called group 1 and the bottom 100 group 2, few people want to abandon group 2 entirely.

Sometimes, unwillingness to abandon patients depends on whether people believe their decision has been made explicitly or implicitly. For example, people were given information about a blood test that divided patients into two prognostic groups and made an allocation choice. We then asked if they would prefer to ignore the blood test and randomly distribute the organs to the children. Forty-one percent said they would choose to ignore the information. Of note, this is larger than the 33%, across the five questionnaire versions, who chose to distribute the organs equally between the groups in the original question. Since ignoring prognostic information leads to the same distribution of organs as distributing them equally between the groups, framing the issue as a choice to use or ignore information led to a more egalitarian response than did describing an example in which the children's prognosis was already known.

One study on age-based rationing reinforced the strength of aversion to abandoning groups of patients. Most people agreed that "life extending medical care should be withheld from older patients to save money to help pay for the medical care of younger patients" (Zweibel, Cassel, & Karrison 1993). However, people also felt strongly that age-based rationing should not be imposed upon patients, but instead should be something that patients should volunteer to do. As the authors stated:

Although a majority of Americans seem willing to withhold life prolonging medical care from critically ill older persons . . . few would categorically withhold such care . . . Rather the American public feels that it is the duty of individual patients, old and young alike, to refuse medical care that would serve only to extend life for a short time.

People do not want to make the hard decisions necessary to control health care costs. They think certain allocation criteria are acceptable ways to set health care priorities, but they are unwilling to use them on anything but a voluntary basis.

Can We Make Any Sense Out of People's Values?

Accumulating evidence suggests that people reject CEA as the sole way of allocating scarce health care resources. But this evidence is mixed, since much of it seems to result as much from cognitive biases as from deeply held values. Clearly, we must do more work to see whether people have consistent preferences and whether these preferences will stabilize once people are made aware of cognitive biases. Nevertheless, it seems reasonable to conclude that CEA does not take account of notions of fairness, which people think ought to play a role in this area. Although fairness is nebulous and complex, it clearly has some elements that people want to see reflected in their health care system. After all, a system that looks only to maximize health, even if that means harming a specific racial group, is unlikely to be well received by the public.

Many people would look at the data presented in this chapter and conclude that measuring the general public's allocation preferences is a waste of time. Instead, we should pick the appropriate theory of justice and allocate health care resources accordingly. Proponents of CEA who believe they have a philosophically justifiable allocation system, might hold that any deviation from CEA expressed by the public is merely a cognitive bias. Proponents of other theories of distributive justice might insist that few people in the general public have the time or inclination to comprehend the superiority of their theory. Thus, any survey demonstrating public rejection of their theory really demonstrates public ignorance.

I am not a proponent of any single theory of distributive justice, which I cannot explain by lack of time or inclination, but can blame only on my indecisive nature or my intellectual weakness. Perhaps because I do not advocate a specific theory I am inclined to take public attitudes seriously. Many allocation dilemmas have no simple solutions, and highly trained, intellectually rigorous philosophers would completely disagree with each other about the best solution, for example, about the extent to which severely ill patients deserve treatment priority. In such situations, the public deserves a role.

But how can such preferences be incorporated into policy making? And how can they compete with the quantifiably powerful information provided by CEA?

In the last section of this book, when I discuss the future of cost-effectiveness and health care rationing, I will show how some of the values described in this chapter, which are currently ignored by CEA, could potentially be incorporated into CEA. But I am not ready to discuss the future yet. Instead, we must first understand a current rationing controversy to gain fuller understanding of the strengths and weaknesses of CEA as a guide—the role of individual clinicians in health care rationing.

II

Cost-Effectiveness and Bedside Rationing: Do Two Wrongs Make a Right?

6

The Case Against Bedside Rationing

In a classic episode of the Simpsons, or perhaps a scene from a Mel Brooks movie (I can't remember), Moses is seen struggling down from the mountain carrying three heavy stone tablets. While holding these tablets, he announces: "People of Israel, I've come down from the mountain with these tablets containing God's fifteen . . ." Moses fumbles with the tablets; one of them drops to the ground and shatters into hundreds of pieces. ". . . Er, ten commandments for how to live a good life."

This is purely speculative, but I bet that, somewhere among those five missing commandments, there is one that says, "Physician, thou shalt not ration." The language used in debates about rationing by physicians (commonly referred to as bedside rationing) often takes on an almost biblical tone:

A physician must do all that is permitted on behalf of his patient. (Hiatt 1975)

Physicians are required to do everything that they believe may benefit each patient without regard to cost. (Levinsky 1984)

The physician provider must continue all treatment efforts without regard to society's just demands for conservation of scarce resources. (Griffin & Thomasma 1983)

The tone of these commentators and nearly all opponents of bedside rationing is one of moral absoluteness akin to a biblical commandment. Physicians, according to one medical ethicist, should pursue patients' benefits even if the benefits are "infinitesimal" (Veatch 1981).

Bedside rationing occurs when a physician or other clinician does less than the best for a patient in order to save societal resources. As the above comments show, many people are adamantly opposed to the practice. If rationing must occur, they contend, it should not be done by clinicians taking care of specific patterns, but by health care professionals or others in settings where they are not taking care of specific patients. That way, patients will know that their clinicians are doing everything in their power to help them.

But bedside rationing should not be so readily dismissed. As Oregon's Medicaid plan showed, it is not easy to make explicit administrative decisions about how to ration health care. Moreover, CEA may be better able to guide these decisions for individual clinicians "at the bedside" than for a large health care provider or a state Medicaid program trying to devise a global plan. At the bedside, clinicians can consider the cost-effectiveness of caring for patients and balance that information with other relevant considerations. If they think CEA undervalues treatments directed at severely ill patients, that can influence their interpretation of a CEA involving severe illnesses. Or it can influence how they think about costs when caring for severely ill patients.

Another reason CEA may work well with bedside rationing is that clinicians can consider clinical factors for specific patients that influence the cost-effectiveness of their care. As we have seen, CEA calculates the average cost divided by the average benefit of caring for a category of patients. But most patients are not average. Suppose a CEA showed that cholesterol treatment in a certain group of patients was a bargain at $25,000 per QALY. Suppose further that this CEA accounted for relevant clinical factors influencing the relationship between cholesterol and vascular disease, such as whether the patient has a history of vascular disease or other illness such as diabetes or high blood pressure. Now imagine a clinician taking care of a sixty-year-old man who has elevated cholesterol and who fits the profile of the patients included in this CEA with one exception—he also has advanced prostate cancer. This makes the man's cholesterol treatment significantly less cost effective. If this patient is likely to die within a couple of years because of prostate cancer, cholesterol treatment is much less likely to benefit him.

Whether to start cholesterol treatment in a patient like this is a difficult decision. But to the extent anyone thinks cost-effectiveness information should guide clinical decisions, it seems preferable to provide the information so that clinicians can place it in the context of specific patients, rather than rely on a guideline that assumes every patient is average.

If CEA is flawed, perhaps clinicians (who make a living applying flawed data to complex situations) can use it in ways that reduce its flaws. But they cannot improve CEA if they are forbidden from rationing. If bedside rationing is always wrong, clinicians should not consider cost-effectiveness information when caring for specific patients.

In this chapter I explore the moral problems with bedside rationing. In subsequent chapters I debate why, despite these problems, it should play a role in how we ration health care.

Moral Problems with Bedside Rationing

Bedside Rationing Involves Rationing

It is no surprise that many people who oppose bedside rationing do so on the grounds that *all* rationing is unjustifiable. I will not revisit this topic. Clearly, if rationing is always wrong, then so is bedside rationing. I have stated that health care rationing is not always wrong. If I have not convinced you that rationing is sometimes necessary and justifiable, I will not convince you that bedside rationing is necessary or justifiable. But, assuming rationing is sometimes justifiable, why do some people think it should never be done by clinicians at the bedside?

Bedside Rationing Violates Clinicians' Advocacy Duties

Patients and clinicians, especially physicians, form a moral relationship that goes beyond that of most professionals and clients. Patients often come to physicians in stressful, compromising situations. They usually rely on physicians to give them advice and counseling regarding their options, and to help them understand their clinical situation. They often feel vulnerable because of their illness (Pellegrino 1979). Sometimes they must reveal intimate secrets so that physicians can diagnose and treat them.

Physicians' moral duties are frequently compared with those of lawyers. People often come to both seeking help in serious circumstances with major life significance. They depend on both for help and they expect both to advocate for their interests. Lawyers and physicians have a great deal of knowledge that brings clients and patients to them in times of need. With such knowledge and power come moral duties.

In fact, many other professions should take their moral duties more seriously. Many people feel powerless when they go to auto mechanics, because they do not know enough about their car engines to tell whether the mechanics are promoting their best interests. What auto mechanics do, of course, does not carry the kind of significance for our lives as what lawyers and physicians do, but there are many ways that the ethics of these professions overlap. (In fact, Mark Siegler teaches University of Chicago medical students about informed consent with the help of an auto mechanic!) The moral duties of any profession escalate in proportion to the knowledge gap between the professionals and their clients, and to the vulnerability of people requesting help. By this measure, physicians' advocacy duties ought to be taken very seriously.

Because physicians have knowledge that is crucial in helping people struggle through important events, they are given special power by society: to prescribe medicines and to cut open people's bodies (with their permission, of course). With this knowledge and power comes a duty to advocate for patients' interests. Any decision to stray from absolute patient advocacy must be done with great caution and with significant moral justification.

Bedside Rationing Will Destroy the Trust Necessary for a Good Doctor-Patient Relationship

Some believe bedside rationing will adversely affect the trust necessary for a good doctor-patient relationship (Hiatt 1975; Pellegrino 1979; Sulmasy 1992). Trust is crucial to the relationship because without it, patients will be less forthcoming in discussing their problems, making it harder for physicians to provide appropriate care. If patients are not forthcoming about their sexual histories, physicians will not know whether they are at risk for sexually transmitted diseases. If patients are unwilling to talk about their alcohol intake, it will have similar consequences.

According to opponents, patients will not trust physicians who ration from them. Because physicians have more knowledge than patients about clinical issues, patients have learned to trust physicians to recommend what is best for them, or to describe the risks and benefits of treatment alternatives in ways that will help them decide what is best for themselves. If physicians ration care, patients will no longer know how to interpret their recommendations: did the physician recommend conservative treatment to help me, or to save money?

Lack of Training about Rationing

Opponents point out that physicians (and other clinicians) have not been trained how to ration health care appropriately. In fact, given general opposition to rationing, and to bedside rationing in particular, physicians have traditionally been taught that they should never do it.

Physicians do, however, have experience balancing patients' best interests with societal interests. For example, they are taught to breach patient confidentiality if there is a public health risk to maintaining confidence. Some states require physicians to report certain infectious diseases to health departments in violation of patient confidentiality. Legal decisions have held that psychiatrists and other health professionals have a duty to breach confidentiality when the patient is a threat to someone else. In addition, physicians have been taught to think about the public health consequences of how they administer antibiotics. They are frequently reminded that broad-spectrum antibiotics should be reserved only for serious, life-threatening infections, or for cases of known resistance to less broad-spectrum antibiotics. Pressure to withhold the drugs is exerted to minimize the development of antibiotic resistance. In many cases this means physicians withhold the best treatment from a patient to decrease (immeasurably but crucially) the long-term risks of resistance to society at large.

Although physicians have been trained to think about public health, they have not been trained to think about public finances. Therefore, asking them to withhold potentially beneficial medical care from patients because it will save money for society is asking them to go beyond their medical expertise.

Bedside Rationing Will Be Discriminatory

Bedside rationing is criticized by some as being vulnerable to discrimination (Macklin 1993). If physicians are told that it is acceptable, they may disproportionately withhold services from patients of certain races or socioeconomic groups. Similarly, the practice is prone to random variability that, although not necessarily discriminatory, raises serious ethical concerns (Sulmasy 1992; Wolf 1994). Some physicians are more likely than others to withhold marginally beneficial care. Thus patients' choice of physician might affect whether they receive certain health care services. Those patients aware of this variability will be at an advantage because they will be more aggressive about obtaining such services.

Physicians, like everyone else, are susceptible to conscious or subconscious biases. Even in Veterans Administration medical centers, where they have no financial incentive to treat poor patients differently than wealthy ones, African-Americans receive fewer cardiovascular procedures than Caucasians, even after adjusting for severity of illnesses (Whittle et al. 1993). Although it is not clear whether this difference is better or worse, since a good chance exists that patients undergo too many of these procedures, and although it is also plausible that patient preferences play some role in who has what test, this difference raises the possibility that subtle racial biases can influence clinical decisions. In fact, even if performing fewer cardiovascular procedures in African-Americans turns out to be clinically advantageous, it could be a good result for a bad reason. Most physicians think that an aggressive approach helps their patients. To the extent they offer more of these procedures to whites than to blacks, we have to be worried about how race can influence clinical decision making.

Discrimination can often be subtle. In one study, physicians allowed longer intervals between visits for obese outpatients than for similarly ill nonobese outpatients. Whether this reflects intention or not is unclear. When supervising residents in outpatient clinics, I have found that some residents give more frequent return visits to patients of whom they are fond: "I really like this guy. I'm going to see him again next month." It is amusing that residents think they are doing patients a favor by seeing them again so soon, but it is also disturbing that this could lead to different health care for patients they like. Most of these residents, and most clinicians in general, would bristle at the thought that they discriminate against patients they do not like. But discrimination does not have to involve conscious decisions to give less care (or worse care) to patients one does not like; it can also result because clinicians give more care (or better care) to patients they do like.

The Savings Brought by Bedside Rationing May not Go to Patients

Some experts argue that bedside rationing is wrong because it creates savings that are not guaranteed to benefit other patients (Cassel 1985; Daniels 1987; Reitemeier & Brody 1988; Wolf 1994). We cannot know, for example, whether the money saved on a low-yield diagnostic test will be used to provide health care goods that are more beneficial, such as childhood vaccines or prenatal care. Savings instead may go toward other health services that bring less benefit, or, worse yet, toward insurance company profits. If physicians ration from their patients, the money they save may simply fatten someone's already-bulging wallet, perhaps even their own. Worse yet, it is maintained, the savings may not even go toward health care; for all we know, they could go toward nonmedical services. Money saved by Medicare could help the government spend money on farm subsidies or the military.

Alternatives to Bedside Rationing: How Opponents Would Ration Health Care

Many people who oppose bedside rationing still believe that some kind of health care rationing is necessary, and they must therefore find other ways to achieve it. In the previous chapter I discussed a number of ways to reduce or eliminate the economic impact of moral hazard. These alternatives shift the locus of rationing from health care professionals, be they clinicians at the bedside or administrators, to patients.

Because these opponents do not think the burden should be shifted completely to patients by increasing their out-of-pocket costs, they prefer alternative mechanisms that do not rely on physicians or patients to make such decisions at the bedside. Three such alternatives are formulary committees, utilization reviewers, and third-party payer reimbursement decisions.

Formulary Committees

Formulary committees decide which drugs will be included in a hospital's or health care system's pharmacy (Fins 1998; Sloan, Gordon, & Cocks 1993). In part, they determine whether new agents are medically effective and appropriate for the institution's patients. But often they make economic decisions such as whether an expensive new drug to treat stomach ulcers is *worth* adding to the formulary, given that a less expensive (and slightly less effective) one is available. In effect, formulary committees sometimes make cost-worthiness judgments.

When a committee decides against adding an expensive new agent to the formulary, clinicians' hands are tied. For example, currently, the Department of Veterans Affairs does not pay for Viagra to treat impotent veterans. Moreover, clinicians practicing solely in VA settings who do not have malpractice insurance to care for non-VA patients are personally liable for adverse events caused by Viagra they prescribe. Thus, many VA physicians have essentially been forbidden from prescribing the drug. Thus they do not have to make cost-worthiness judgments about Viagra, if they were ever inclined to do so, because that decision has been made for them.

Utilization Review

Utilization reviewers and case managers determine whether patients require hospitalization or expensive testing. For example, sometimes clinicians must obtain authorization from a case manager before hospitalizing a patient or ordering an MRI scan. Other times a reviewer visits a hospitalized patient and notifies the hospital team that the insurance company will not pay for a longer stay. Once again, as with the formulary committee decision, utilization reviewer decisions tie clinicians' hands. In these cases, the reviewers make the rationing decisions, thereby freeing clinicians from the need do it.

Reimbursement Decisions

At a higher level, governments and health care systems can make rationing decisions by limiting services physicians may provide. Governments administer certificate of need laws to limit the amount of expensive new technology available to physicians and patients (Furrow 1988). Although these laws have not succeeded in limiting technology diffusion (Bryce & Cline 1998), in theory they could make some services less available, thereby relieving physicians of the job of rationing health care. Physicians who cannot order a PET scan cannot be accused of rationing the scan.

Similarly, insurance companies and managed care organizations can decide whether to pay for specific treatments.

For a while, most managed care organizations did not pay for bone marrow transplantation in women with metastatic breast cancer. Physicians who thought that a transplant was necessary were precluded from offering this treatment, or were required to provide it without reimbursement. After several lawsuits, bone marrow transplantation is universally covered, despite lack of compelling evidence that it works. But that is another story (Anders 1996).

Oregon's rationing plan is another example of a reimbursement decision that relieved clinicians of the need to ration. If Medicaid won't pay for a service, physicians cannot be blamed for withholding it.

Common to these alternative mechanisms is that they withhold beneficial services *before* patients interact with physicians. Thus, they do not rely on physicians to ration at the bedside. Instead, they tie physicians' hands so that they cannot provide certain services. This allows physicians to avoid rationing and lets them promote patients' best interests by offering them the best services *available*.

Not All Administrative Efforts to Decrease Costs Avoid Bedside Rationing

Opponents of bedside rationing champion many administrative rationing mechanisms. However, this does not mean that all administrative efforts to decrease costs avoid bedside rationing. In fact, many of them rely on bedside rationing to succeed. For example, insurance companies and managed care organizations have adopted practice guidelines, clinical pathways, capitation payments, and feedback mechanisms to decrease resource use. All of these mechanisms rely on bedside rationing.

Practice Guidelines and Clinical Pathways

Practice guidelines and clinical pathways attempt to make physicians practice medicine in a more consistent manner (Brook 1989; Weingarten et al. 1994). The main reason that they were developed is to reduce unacceptable variations in physician's clinical decisions. For example, the rate for hysterectomy in the United States varies depending on what area a woman lives in (Wennberg & Gittelsohn 1982). This suggests that many unnecessary hysterectomies are being performed. Practice guidelines attempt to help physicians determine when such a procedure is indicated. Similarly, clinical pathways attempt to make patients' hospital stays more consistent, predictable, and perhaps medically justifiable. For example, a clinical pathway might recommend that a patient who has bypass surgery should be up and walking on postoperative day 3.

Although these approaches are designed primarily to improve health care quality, they are also used to ration marginally beneficial health care. A clinical pathway that recommends discharging a patient five days after surgery may in part reflect a belief that the additional cost of day 6 is not worth the expense.

If practice guidelines and clinical pathways are ever to succeed as rationing tools, physicians must be willing to follow them. They are *guidelines*, after all, not rules. Clinical pathways help physicians take care of typical patients, but physicians have the discretion to decide when to deviate from them. A physician who thinks all patients would benefit from six days of hospitalization after surgery, instead of the five recommended by a practice guideline, can simply keep each patient in the hospital for six days.

Other cost control (and quality improvement) mechanisms, such as computer reminder systems that reduce the use of expensive drugs (McDonald et al. 1996) and feedback reports that tell physicians how their resource use compares with that of other physicians (Berwick & Coltin 1986; Schectman, Elinsky, & Pawlson 1991; Spiegel et al. 1989; Winikoff et al. 1984), may reduce physicians' resource use by encouraging bedside rationing. It is surprising how little attention has been given to these forms of rationing. If physicians are reminded by computers or feedback reports that they are prescribing expensive drugs, they prescribe less expensive alternatives. Whereas some of these less expensive agents are equally effective as more expensive ones, they are often inferior. In such cases, a reminder to prescribe the less expensive one encourages bedside rationing.

Capitation Arrangements

Managed care organizations in the United States (Hillman et al. 1991; Hillman 1987, 1990; Hillman, Pauly, & Kerstein 1989) and more recently in the United Kingdom (Klein 1998) attempt to decrease costs by paying clinicians according to capitation arrangements. Capitation is a reimbursement mechanism that is best understood by contrasting it with traditional fee-for-service methods under which health care providers are paid according to what they do for patients. For a fifteen-minute visit, they receive a certain amount of money; for a thirty-minute visit they receive more. Clinicians (or health systems) receive additional money for each laboratory test ordered, each procedure performed, and each additional day patients remain in the hospital. Under fee-for-service, the more you do, the more you are paid.

Under capitation, clinicians or health systems are paid a lump sum for each patient they care for, and tests and procedures they order come out of this pot. Thus clinicians are *at risk* for health care expenses that go beyond what they have been paid. If a physician receives $100 a month to care for a patient, anything she spends beyond that is her loss, and everything less is her gain. For that reason, capitation has been heavily criticized by many people who believe that physicians should not have incentives to do less for patients. Whatever one thinks of capitation, however, clearly it only works by encouraging bedside rationing.

In short, practice guidelines, clinical pathways, computer reminders, feedback reports, and capitations arrangements are formal mechanisms devised by hospitals, health care systems, and other higher-level parties to encourage physicians to decrease resource use even to the point of bedside rationing. If physicians refuse to do this, all of these arrangements will not decrease health care costs.

Summary

In this chapter I outlined the main reasons why most experts are opposed to bedside rationing: it violates physicians' advocacy duties, damages the trust inherent in the doctor-patient relationship, requires physicians to do something they are not trained to do, creates the possibility for discrimination, and does not provide savings that are guaranteed to improve health. In response to these serious (and largely accurate) criticisms, health care institutions and others have developed several alternatives including government or third-party payer mechanisms that reduce the availability of services to physicians and patients, and institutional administrative mechanisms such as formulary committees and utilization review. Ultimately, I maintain that these mechanisms are insufficient, and that health care rationing will succeed only if physicians relax their advocacy duties occasionally (cautiously and carefully) to ration at the bedside.

7

Recognizing Bedside Rationing

A physician prescribes antibiotics for a woman with classic symptoms of a urinary tract infection, but does not order a bacterial culture of her urine.

An orthopedic surgeon places a particular artificial hip prosthesis into a seventy-eight-year-old woman, even though a prosthesis made by another company is known to last longer.

A nephrologist orders dialysis for patients for an average of nine hours a week, even though longer dialysis times provide patients with better quality of life.

A family practitioner refers a patient to a vascular surgeon in the patient's health plan, even though a world-renowned vascular surgeon is just around the corner.

These are common examples that many physicians encounter on a daily basis. Given the moral problems associated with bedside rationing, it is important to know whether these physicians are rationing care from their patients. When does a physician's decision to do less than the best for a patient qualify as bedside rationing?

It is useless to debate the issue without a clear understanding of what it takes for a clinician's decision to qualify as bedside rationing. A series of cases illustrate the process.

Agreeing on a Definition

According to the definition stated earlier, three conditions must be met before a clinician's actions qualify as bedside rationing. The clinician must:

1. withhold, withdraw or fail to recommend a service that, in the clinician's best judgment, is in the patient's best medical interests;

2. act primarily to promote the financial interest of someone other than the patient, including an organization, society at large, or the clinician himself or herself, and

3. have control over the use of the medically beneficial service.

An example helps show what types of actions qualify as bedside rationing:

Streptokinase or TPA? Joe arrives at the local emergency room with classic signs and symptoms of a heart attack. He feels like an elephant is sitting on his chest, making it hard to breath and making him seriously fear that he will not live through the night. The emergency room resident, Dr. Carter, decides to treat him with Streptokinase (SK), a clot-busting drug that helps limit the damage caused by a heart attack. Dr. Carter chooses SK rather than tissue plasminogen activator (TPA), even though TPA is slightly better for this type of heart attack. A course of TPA costs over $1,000, and Dr. Carter thinks the incremental benefits over SK are not worth the additional cost. Joe is unaware of this decision and only hopes that Dr. Carter will do everything in his power to save his life and put an end to his intense pain.

This is an example of bedside rationing, because Dr. Carter withheld a service that would have been in Joe's best medical interests; TPA is a better treatment for Joe than SK (GUSTO, 1993). In addition, Dr. Carter had control over the resource and was withholding it out of a desire to save money for society, thereby placing society's financial interests ahead of Joe's best medical interests.

Why This Definition?

The definition of bedside rationing is based on a review of the literature pertaining to debates about the morality of the practice in which these three components are implicit in people's opposition or support. Marcia Angell (1993), in opposing bedside rationing, stated that "anything short of full efforts to heal the individual patient, then, must involve a hidden agenda—an ethically indefensible position." Robert Veatch (1981), quoted in the previous chapter, said that physicians have to pursue care that is "even infinitesimally beneficial to the patient." Marsh and Yarborough (1990) stated, "It is inconceivable morally that a physician can act in the patient's best interests while . . . promoting the economic welfare of the institution he represents."

Whereas few discussions of bedside rationing have proposed explicit definitions (Levinsky 1998), implicit is the notion that doing anything less than the best for patients to save money for society constitutes bedside rationing. These are two of the three conditions: (1) a beneficial service must be withheld from patients (2) to save societal resources. The third condition, that the clinician should have control over this resource, is also implicit. After all, if physicians have no control over the use of a resource, they cannot be accused of doing the rationing.

Some may wonder whether withholding infinitesimal benefits from patients really constitutes bedside rationing. Strictly speaking, if a benefit is infinitesimal, it is nonexistent, and no one questions the appropriateness of withholding nonexistent benefits. However, in mentioning infinitesimal benefits, Veatch points out that rationing occurs when clinicians withhold even the very tiniest of benefits, and he is correct. First, any other cut-off would be arbitrary. After all, if we contend that withholding very small benefits does not constitute bedside rationing, how much benefit has to exist before something is rationing? Second, moral debates on the topic center on advocacy duties—just how far should clinicians go to advocate for patients' best interests? Once they start withholding even tiny benefits they have begun to relax their advocacy duties. Because these debates are essentially about whether clinicians' advocacy duties for individual patients are ever limited by society's financial interests, withholding *any* amount of benefit is the best point at which to say that a clinician is rationing at the bedside.

Am I up to my shenanigans again? Have I stacked the deck in my favor by defining bedside rationing so broadly that everyone would have to agree that it is inevitable and appropriate? I don't think so. After all, respected people such as Marcia Angell (1985), Arnold Relman (1990b), and Robert Veatch (1981), among others, have argued that clinicians' advocacy duties are absolute. Norman Levinsky (1998), a respected medical leader and scholar, adopted the above definition of bedside rationing at the same time as he reaffirmed his strong opposition to the practice.

Although the definition used in this book is fair, I also want to make sure it is clear. With that purpose in mind, I provide a series of cases to illustrate the three conditions of bedside rationing. Many examples *fail* to meet one or more of the conditions, thus elucidating the importance of each condition.

Recognizing Bedside Rationing: Illustrative Cases

Condition 1: Health Care Services Are Withheld that Are in Patients' Best Interests

Before an act can qualify as bedside rationing, it must qualify as rationing. In chapter 2, I defined health care rationing as any implicit or explicit mechanism that allows people to go without beneficial health care services. In this chapter, I defined the first condition of bedside rationing as withholding a service that is in the patient's best medical interests. Thus, the condition determines whether rationing has occurred. (The second and third conditions, which are discussed in more detail below, determine whether the rationing qualifies as *bedside* rationing.) The importance of the first condition is illustrated by the following case.

Treatment of Mild Hypertension   Mr. Nye, an otherwise healthy 46-year-old, is diagnosed by Dr. Neff as having mild high blood pressure. He has been dieting and exercising for six months, but his blood pressure is still elevated. Dr. Neff prescribes generic hydrochlorothiazide (HCTZ), a water pill that lowers blood pressure. Dr. Neff is chided by her colleagues for suggesting this old, inexpensive drug when newer ones are available. Dr. Neff is uncomfortable knowing that she prefers this older agent in part because it is less expensive.

At first glance, this appears to be bedside rationing: Dr. Neff prescribes HCTZ rather than some new blood pressure-lowering drug because it is less expensive. However, although she considered costs, she did not ration at the bedside, because the newer, more expensive alternatives are not any better at controlling mild hypertension than HCTZ (Alderman 1992; Moser 1993). Nor do they have better side effect profiles.

It is easy to imagine a change in this case that would make it meet the first condition of bedside rationing. If Mr. Nye was diabetic, an angiotensin-converting enzyme inhibitor, one of a more expensive class of antihypertensive agents would benefit him more than HCTZ because of its beneficial effects on kidney function (Viberti et al. 1994). But Mr. Nye has no other health problems, and thus Dr. Neff's choice of the less expensive drug does not sacrifice his best interests. Dr. Neff should not be uncomfortable for considering costs. Instead, she should recognize that she eliminated waste by offering an equally beneficial and less expensive therapy.

Clinicians should eliminate waste whenever possible. Considering costs when services are of equal benefit is morally praiseworthy in that it can help provide other necessary services in the context of limited resources without additional burdens. *Factoring costs into treatment decisions is not necessarily rationing.*

Although eliminating waste is an admirable goal, it is not always easy to know which medical options are in patients' best interests. As discussed in chapter 2, many health care services have not been proved to be better or worse than others. Whether withholding them qualifies as rationing is a judgment call.

Clinicians themselves may differ in their skepticism for new treatments, their judgments about evidence, and their assessment of the importance of the patient's medical interests. Thus, judgments of benefit are likely to vary. A caution, however, is in order, as illustrated in the next case.

The PSA Test   Mr. Jordan, a 60-year-old man with no significant medical problems, visits his primary care physician and asks whether he should have the PSA test, saying, "My closest friend was just diagnosed with prostate cancer and has it all over his body. I'd rather go through anything than have that happen to me." Mr. Jordan has no signs or symptoms suggestive of prostate cancer. His physician describes the risks and benefits of the PSA test and the controversy surrounding it. And although he knows several urologists and primary care physicians who routinely perform the test, he thinks its risks outweigh the benefits. The physician convinces Mr. Jordan to go without the PSA blood test.

The PSA test is not proved to prevent people from dying of prostate cancer. On the other hand, it does detect the disease earlier than digital rectal examination (Collins & Barry 1996). Until adequate trials are completed, this is a case of reasonable people being able to disagree about whether the glass is half full or half empty. Many people are ardent advocates of the test, whereas others feel it causes unnecessary biopsies and worries.

Some clinicians may find that the psychological benefits of the PSA test warrant it in some patients, even if most men would not benefit from it. Where reasonable clinicians disagree, patients' preferences may influence whether services are medically beneficial (Ubel 1996; Wolf et al. 1996). Suppose Mr. Jordan was unusually tense about his risk of prostate cancer. A clinician may decide that the PSA test is warranted to put him at ease. Here, of course, the clinician must consider the anxiety a false positive result would create. If the patient's PSA level is high, even if he does not have prostate cancer, he could suffer before the disease is ruled out.

In determining the benefits of specific health care services, clinicians have to evaluate the services from the patient's perspective (Barry et al. 1988; Pauker & McNeil 1981). Refusing to authorize a test, even if the patient bears the cost, abuses the power discrepancy in the clinician-patient relationship and fails to respect patients' values and goals. To prevent the patient's perspective from overwhelming all judgments of clinical effectiveness, however, patients' requests should fit within the range of reasonable medical opinion (Brett & McCullough 1986). Where consensus exists about the potential benefits of a particular service (for example, when a national panel of experts strongly supports a less expensive antihypertension agent), requests for another service should be accorded less weight. Similarly, when potential harm clearly and uncontroversially outweighs benefits (for example, exercise stress tests for young, asymptomatic women), this is not bedside rationing, because the decision is based on balancing risks and benefits, not on cost considerations.

Considering costs is thus a necessary, but not sufficient, condition for bedside rationing. Also necessary is the judgment that a medical benefit (valued by the patient) is being withheld. Despite difficulty knowing what the best alternative is, the moral point remains straightforward. Bedside rationing does not occur unless there is good reason, based on the clinician's best judgment and including attention to the patient's preferences and values, to think that the patient has not received a medically beneficial service. One way to determine whether a decision is based on patients' preferences, medical risks and benefits, or society's financial interests is for clinicians to ask themselves, "Would I be willing to provide or authorize this service if it were free, or if patients were paying for it themselves?" In this way, cases in which harms outweigh benefits can be separated from those in which benefits are not worth the costs.

Condition 2: The Clinician Acts Primarily to Promote the Financial Interests of Someone Other than the Patient

According to condition 1, cases qualify as examples of health care rationing when a service is withheld that would have been in the patient's best medical interests. In such cases, conditions 2 and 3 help determine whether the rationing is an example of bedside rationing or some other form. The following case illustrates the importance of this condition.

Antibiotic Treatment of a Urinary Tract Infection   Over the past 36 hours, Ms. Baron has been in and out of the bathroom, and every time she urinates, it causes intense burning pain. She has classic symptoms of a urinary tract infection (UTI). Her physician orders a urinalysis, which reveals white blood cells and many bacteria, confirming the presence of a UTI. Ms. Baron has no known allergies, but has not taken any sulfa drugs before. Her physician prescribes three days of trimethoprim-sulfamethoxazole, an inexpensive sulfa antibiotic that successfully cures 90% of UTIs. Her physician does this even though ciprofloxacin, an expensive, powerful, broad-spectrum antibiotic, would have a better chance of curing her and a smaller risk of side effects (Grubbs et al. 1992). The physician is aware of concerns about increasing antibiotic resistance to ciprofloxacin, which is often critical in treating life-threatening infections.

This case meets the first condition of bedside rationing. It does not, however, meet the second. The physician did not withhold ciprofloxacin primarily for *financial* reasons, but to prevent development of resistance to this important agent. To maintain the effectiveness of broad-spectrum antibiotics in severe illnesses, it is necessary to administer less potent antibiotics for common conditions such as the one afflicting Ms. Baron (Lipsitch 1995). Thus, as this case shows, the second condition of bedside rationing is important because many decisions physicians make are meant to promote public health or other important objectives, rather than to promote the financial interests of someone other than their patients. These decisions do not qualify as bedside rationing because they balance nonmonetary goods and harms accruing to others against the medical benefit to the patient. Instead, they qualify as other forms of health care rationing.

The choice of ciprofloxacin is an example of noneconomic rationing, in which the patient does not receive the best medical treatment because of some nonfinancial reason; in this case, to promote public health. Another example is allocation of scarce transplant organs where decisions could be made to withhold organs from some patients who are not as likely to benefit as others (Ubel et al. 1993).

These examples of noneconomic rationing are still fraught with moral complexities, many of which are also associated with bedside rationing. I have chosen to exclude noneconomic rationing primarily to be consistent with how bedside rationing is debated in the literature. Physicians have universally been encouraged to think about public health risks when they prescribe antibiotics. At the same time, they have largely been discouraged from bedside rationing. Thus, noneconomic rationing traditionally has not counted as bedside rationing. In addition, it does not carry all the moral problems associated with bedside rationing. Specifically, physicians are trained to conduct noneconomic rationing and are not trained to conduct economic rationing.

Nevertheless, I would be willing to broaden the definition of bedside rationing I use here to include noneconomic rationing. But those who oppose bedside rationing would disagree with such broadening, since it would incorporate traditionally acceptable rationing decisions. If the definition was broadened to include cases such as Ms. Baron's, almost no one would be opposed to it. The definition would then distort debates about bedside rationing in which opponents almost always object to clinicians' considerations of society's financial interests. Thus, in the remainder of this book, I continue to use a narrower definition that excludes cases in which patients' best interests are sacrificed solely to promote public health concerns.

Out-of-Pocket Antihistamine Costs Andrea, a 20-year-old college student, comes to the college walk-in clinic with symptoms of seasonal allergic rhinitis, that sneezy, itchy, sniffly feeling when ragweed invades fragile sinus cavities. The physician discusses treatment options with her and recommends a trial of antihistamines. He mentions that inexpensive over-the-counter antihistamines are often effective for allergy symptoms, but cause drowsiness in some people. More expensive ones do not cause drowsiness. Because Andrea has no prescription coverage, she asks to try the less expensive antihistamine first.

This is an example of economic rationing that does not qualify as bedside rationing. Although cost was a factor in this physician's prescription decision, it is clear that the decision was made primarily to promote Andrea's financial interests by reducing her out-of-pocket expenses. Patients' interests are not purely medical; when treatment decisions have a financial impact, their interests are affected in nonmedical ways. In addition, in this case, the decision was made primarily by Andrea; the physician explained the relative merits and demerits of alternatives, and she weighed the cost-worthiness of the more expensive medication using her own valuation of costs and benefits. Thus, this is a rationing decision with the more beneficial antihistamine rationed according to willingness to pay. But this is not bedside rationing, because the physician did not withhold the more expensive antihistamine to serve someone's financial interests other than the patient's.

One can imagine a variation in which the physician prescribed a less expensive drug without discussing the more expensive alternative. Even though the physician may have been motivated by the patient's financial interests, it would be unclear whether those interests had been served, because some patients might be willing to spend more money to avoid possible sedation. The only way to discover this is to discuss alternatives with the patient. Similarly, patients often make their own rationing decisions about services available only at a great geographic distance. Here their costs of travel and inconvenience may tip the balance against an otherwise medically beneficial service. When patients care about costs, such discussions are an integral and important part of informed consent (Ubel & Loewenstein 1997).

If Andrea had not had out-of-pocket expenses, or had had a copay that did not vary with the cost of the drug, and if the physician had offered only the less expensive choice without discussing the alternative, it would have been a clear example of bedside rationing. The physician would have judged that the additional benefit of the more expensive drug was not worth the extra cost to society. When the patient makes the value judgment, it is not bedside rationing; only when a clinician does can it qualify as bedside rationing.

Dan Sulmasy, an ethicist and general internist, maintains that physicians' decisions to withhold care from patients to serve someone else's financial interests do not always qualify as bedside rationing. Specifically, when physicians withhold beneficial services to increase their own salaries, such as when they are paid through capitation arrangements, their decisions are examples of greed.

It is correct that greed can cause physicians to withhold benefits from patients. But, surely, acting greedily does not disqualify an action from being an example of rationing. Bedside rationing can also be motivated by altruism. Physicians working in a fee-for-service environment may withhold a beneficial service to save money for society, even though their incomes will be slightly reduced.

The three conditions of bedside rationing proposed here are meant to be morally neutral—they do not signify whether rationing is moral or immoral, appropriate or inappropriate, greedy or altruistic. For those who think it is always inappropriate, these conditions help identify acts all clinicians should avoid. For those who think it is sometimes appropriate, the conditions allow clinicians to reflect on whether a particular instance is morally appropriate.

Condition 3: The Clinician Has Control Over Use of the Medically Beneficial Service

Hospital Control of Contrast Agents   Dr. Carlson tells Mr. Olsen that the best way to evaluate his urinary problems is with an intravenous pyelogram (IVP) film of his kidneys. He explains that Mr. Olsen will be injected with a contrast dye to help radiologists visualize his urinary tract. In this case, Mr. Olsen is injected with a high-osmolar contrast agent and experiences uncomfortable nausea. High-osmolar contrast agents are the traditional dyes used for IVPs. Later, Mr. Olsen learns that low-osmolar contrast agents are less likely to cause this uncomfortable side effect (Steinberg et al. 1992). Dr. Carlson is sorry that Mr. Olsen experienced the side effect, but hospital policy precludes him from ordering low-osmolar contrast agents unless patients are known to be at high risk of a serious adverse reaction.

This case meets the first condition of bedside rationing—a service is withheld that would have been in the patient's best medical interests. It also meets the second condition, because the policy is in place to conserve societal (or hospital) resources (Eddy 1992a). However, it does not meet the third condition. This physician does not have control over use of the low-osmolar contrast agent; instead, the *hospital* limited the use of the better, but more expensive, contrast agent.

Rationing often occurs at levels other than individual clinician-patient encounters. Formulary committees, utilization reviewers, and third-party payers can all limit clinicians' actions. Clinicians may even play crucial roles as sources of information or expertise in these organizational decisions. For example, many clinicians sit on hospital formulary committees. Although formulary committee members should think about the moral implications of their decisions (Hochla & Tuason 1992), clinician members are not bound by the same moral duties as when they are working directly with patients. Clinicians can also participate in designing rationing plans, such as Oregon's Medicaid experiment, without being accused of rationing at the bedside. Those who limit the use of expensive drugs through formulary committees are making population-based, organizational-level rationing judgments that may at some point influence what is available for individual patients. Similarly, clinicians creating government or organization rationing policies are not rationing at the bedside.

Use of Scarce MRI Slots   Dr. Decker works at a county hospital without an MRI scanner. The hospital puts money aside each year for six patients to have MRIs at a nearby hospital. Dr. Decker is evaluating Mr. Dylan who has a "soft indication" for an MRI. He could send Mr. Dylan for an MRI. However, he knows that by doing so he prevents another patient from having the MRI who possibly needs it more. Thus, he tells Mr. Dylan that an MRI is not necessary.

At first glance, this case does not appear to be bedside rationing. It is not, one might insist, the price of the MRI that is preventing Dr. Decker from ordering it, but the scarcity of time slots, the "absolute scarcity" of this service. He also does not appear to have control over the service, since the hospital limits the number of yearly MRIs. However, these appearances are deceptive. In fact it *is* Dr. Decker who decides when and whether to order the MRI, and thus has control at the individual decision-making level. The decision indirectly conserves services (scarce MRI slots) in the interests of other, presumably needier patients. Although it is not dollars per se being saved, restrictions on the numbers of services, or intensive care beds, or staff, are made ultimately for financial reasons. Money is, after all, merely the medium of exchange for all health care (and other) resources.

One could contend that these MRI slots, like intensive care beds or solid organs, are an absolute scarce resource, whereas money is a relatively scarce one. This distinction, however, is a false dichotomy (Morreim 1985). Resources are *always* limited. They may be stringently limited, as in this case, or more gently limited, if, for instance this hospital had its own MRI scanner and thus could scan hundreds of patients per year.

Thus, withholding and not recommending a potentially beneficial MRI counts as bedside rationing. It may be morally justified, but should not be dismissed as a noneconomic decision. This example illustrates the importance of economic honesty. Only openness about these sorts of choices will allow society to debate the merits and morality of these issues.

Clear Cases and Tough Calls

As these cases illustrate, the calls are tough and often subtle when trying to decide whether a clinical decision qualifies as bedside rationing. It is not always easy to know what is in patients' best medical interests. Medical data on risks and benefits of many services are frequently unclear, and assessment of evidence is itself a value-laden process. Nor is it easy to know what is in patients' best financial interests if patients do not know their copayment responsibilities.

Although there will always be tough cases, it is helpful for clinicians to be able to recognize when their actions definitely do or do not qualify as bedside rationing. It is also important for those debating the moral question to be able to recognize these acts. Figure 7.1 summarizes three questions that help identify them.

Question 1: Would it have been in the patient's best medical interests to receive the service being withheld? When a service is withheld that is not in patients' best medical interests, no rationing of any type is occurring, bedside or other. If the service would clearly have been in the patient's best medical interests, the case involves some form of health care rationing, bedside or other. When it is unclear what is in the patient's best medical interests, it is also unclear whether rationing is involved. Then it is reasonable to ask the next two questions, illustrated in figure

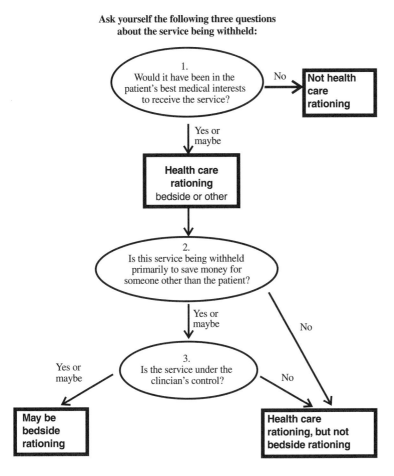

Figure 7.1
How to recognize when withholding a service might qualify as bedside rationing.
(Reprinted from Ubel & Gold 1997.)

7.1. It is better to err on the side of overidentifying cases of bedside rationing, so that one can decide whether it is justifiable to withhold services.

Question 2: Is the service being withheld primarily to save money for someone other than the patient? If clinicians are withholding services to promote public health or to pursue other nonmonetary goals, they are not engaged in bedside rationing. Similarly, when a patient chooses a less expensive option because of its costs, rationing is not by the clinician but is self-imposed.

Question 3: Is the service under the clinician's control? If clinicians' use of services is limited by, for example, administrative mechanisms, withholding these services is not an example of bedside rationing but of rationing through administrative mechanisms. If clinicians had complete control over use of the service, the decision to withhold is bedside rationing. In many cases, how much control clinicians have will be unclear. Frequently, clinicians must spend time to obtain approval for a service. At that point, they must decide whether or not to spend that time. But, if it is in their power to advocate for patients and provide the best possible care, a decision *not* to take the necessary time to do this qualifies as bedside rationing.

When the answer to all three questions is "yes," clinicians will have rationed at the bedside. Then they must seriously consider whether their decisions are justified. The medical profession has yet to decide whether bedside rationing is ever morally justified, and, if so, under what circumstances. I propose in chapter 9 that clinicians have an important role in limiting the use of marginally beneficial services because they can account for patients' individual characteristics and preferences, which higher-level rationing mechanisms cannot do. But even I, who do not absolutely oppose bedside rationing, acknowledge its moral problems. Thus, bedside rationing must be done with great caution; key to this caution is the ability to identify it.

When the answer to one or more of the questions is "no," clinicians do not have to worry that they have participated in bedside rationing. When the answer to the questions is "maybe," clinicians may be participating in bedside rationing. They should take these cases very seriously, therefore, and carefully consider whether their decisions are morally justified.

8

Linguistic Confusion about Bedside Rationing

Imagine two people gazing at an insect. They agree that the insect is beautiful, but disagree about whether it is a moth or a butterfly.

Now consider two other people staring at the same insect. These two are in complete agreement that it is a moth, but disagree about whether it is beautiful or ugly.

The first observers agree about their subjective evaluation of the insect, but do not agree on what name to call it. The second pair agree about what to call the insect, but disagree about their subjective evaluation of its beauty or lack thereof.

Similar problems plague debates about bedside rationing. In the previous chapter I discussed three conditions of bedside rationing. Although the conditions make sense, given the way most people debate the morality of bedside rationing, not everyone agrees about how to define it. Because of such disagreements, it may be difficult to distinguish between disagreements about what it means to ration at the bedside and those about the appropriateness of doing so.

Debates about appropriateness are often confounded with linguistic confusion over what it means to ration at the bedside. Data show, in fact, that most physicians think it is appropriate to withhold marginally beneficial services, but most do not want to admit that this qualifies as rationing. Instead, they find other ways of coming to terms with what they are doing. Foregoing a urine culture is not rationing, it is simply "the standard of care." Using a less durable hip prosthesis in a 78-year-old woman certainly cannot qualify as rationing when it is "cost-effective medicine"!

A Survey of General Internists: Exploring Attitudes Toward Rationing and Withholding Beneficial Care

To disentangle the concept from the language, David Asch (a general internist colleague) and I conducted a survey in which we gave general internists case vignettes in which a hypothetical clinician, Dr. Smith, was described as choosing less effective cancer screening tests for two patients. The colon cancer screening vignette was as follows.

Mr. Williams comes to Dr. Smith for a routine physical examination. Mr. Williams is a healthy 55-year-old without a family history of colon cancer. Insurance covers the cost of all diagnostic tests. Patients like Mr. Williams have approximately 1 chance in 100 of developing colon cancer over ten years. Therefore, Dr. Smith decides to test Mr. Williams for colon cancer every ten years, starting now. Two tests are available. Test A costs $100 and detects 90% of colon cancers; test B costs $400 and detects 95%. Dr. Smith chooses test A.

The cervical cancer screening vignette was as follows.

Mrs. Jordan comes to Dr. Smith for a routine physical examination. She is a healthy 44-year-old who has never had an abnormal Pap smear. Insurance covers the cost of all diagnostic tests. Pap smears cost approximately $50. In women like Mrs. Jordan, a Pap smear performed every three years detects 90% of cancers; one performed every year detects 91%. Thus they have have approximately 1 chance in 250 of developing cervical cancer over three years. Dr. Smith tells Mrs. Jordan that he will not do a Pap smear this year, but will instead perform one every three years.

Readers will recognize this last vignette from David Eddy's cost-effectiveness article discussed in the introduction (Eddy 1990). Readers should also recognize that both vignettes qualify as bedside rationing. Dr. Smith withheld the most effective screening tests from both patients and had control over which ones to perform. Although it is not clear why he made those choices, it is implied that it was to save money, because no other reason is given.

David Asch and I chose these vignettes in part because they meet all three conditions of bedside rationing, and also because they are common settings in which such practice occurs in the real world. Screening tests almost always require physicians to think about costs. Textbooks teach that good screening tests should be inexpensive and should detect common and curable diseases (Eddy, 1991a). In short, they should be cost effective. The books rarely discuss morality, but put forth the criteria as medical—not value—judgments. Thus, Asch and I thought that many physicians might make cost-worthiness judgments about screening tests without recognizing them as rationing. We wanted to see whether physicians thought that withholding the best available screening tests was appropriate in these circumstances, and whether doing so would quality as bedside rationing.

For both vignettes we asked physicians how much they agreed (on a seven-point scale ranging from completely disagree to completely agree) that (1) Dr. Smith's choices were appropriate, and (2) that they were examples of health care rationing. In addition, we asked physicians to indicate (on the same scale) how much they agreed with the statement, "I believe that physicians should never ration medical care."

We received completed questionnaires from 528 physicians (55% response) and found general agreement that Dr. Smith acted appropriately, but significant disagreement about whether this constituted rationing (figure 8.1). Responses to the two vignettes were almost identical. Over 70% of physicians agreed that choices for both patients were appropriate, with only 20% disagreeing. On the other hand, opinions were evenly split about whether the choices were examples of health care rationing. Opinions were equally divided about whether "physicians should never ration medical care"; 38% of physicians agreed with this statement and 45% disagreed. The rest were undecided.

A couple of other things were clear from our analysis of the responses. First, physicians who thought that these vignettes were examples of rationing were likely to say that Dr. Smith's actions were inappropriate, as were those who agreed that physicians should never ration medical care. Indeed, for those who said physicians should never ration medical care, the judgments of whether Dr. Smith's actions were viewed as rationing or appropriate were very strongly associated. If they thought Dr. Smith rationed, they generally concluded that his actions were inappropriate. In contrast, for physicians who were not absolute opponents of rationing (in other words, who disagreed with the statement "physicians should never ration medical care"), the association between rationing and appropriateness was much weaker. Whether they classified Dr. Smith's actions as rationing was relatively unassociated with whether they thought his actions were appropriate.

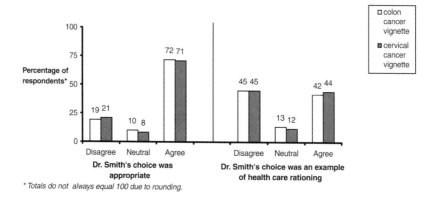

Figure 8.1
Distribution of responses regarding whether Dr. Smith's choices of the less effective cancer screening strategies were appropriate and consisted of rationing.

This changing relationship between rationing judgments and appropriateness judgments makes sense. I classify myself, if not as a proponent of bedside rationing, then as someone who does not absolutely oppose it. I disagree, in other words, that physicians should never ration medical care. So, when I decide whether a case is rationing, this is separate from my decision about whether it is appropriate. I think some rationing is appropriate and some is inappropriate. In contrast, for those who absolutely oppose bedside rationing, the term will be applied only to actions they consider inappropriate. If choosing a less effective screening test feels appropriate, they will not classify it as rationing.

This study reveals broad agreement among general internists that it is appropriate to do less than the best for their patients, especially when additional benefits come at significant financial costs. In the first vignette it would cost approximately $600,000 for each colon cancer detected by the better screening test that would not have been detected by the less effective test (Eddy et al. 1987). This is an incredibly high price, and physicians seem comfortable withholding benefits that come at such great cost. At the same time, many may not be willing to admit that withholding this benefit qualifies as bedside rationing.

If physicians are willing to do less than the best for their patients but are unwilling to agree that this is rationing, how do they reconcile their actions with this view? They simply find other ways to characterize their acts. In the next section I give examples of how physicians think about these types of cases.

Rationing by Any Other Name

Sometimes it is easier to live with ourselves if we don't put a name to our thoughts or actions. I am reminded of a conversation I had with a close friend shortly after she became engaged to an atheist. I have nothing against atheists, but I did express some surprise about my friend's ensuing marriage, given her strong Roman Catholic faith.

"Peter," she said, "I may not be as Catholic as you think."

This was a statement I could not ignore. I questioned her about her faith, starting with an easy question: "Do you believe in a single God who created the world and watches over us?" She did. "Okay. Another easy question. Do you believe that Jesus Christ is both man and God, was killed and rose three days later . . .?"

She cut me off. "Well, that's where I start having some doubts."

I was shocked. I expected we might run into trouble when it came to the Church's view on premarital sex or birth control. But here she was questioning the very basis of Christianity.

"It sounds to me like you're not even Christian!"

My friend was very distressed. She had not yet realized that her changing faith qualified her as a monotheist but not as a Christian. She no longer believed that Christ was anything other than a good moral teacher. She could express her doubts about Christ being God, but was not willing to take on the label of being a non-Christian.

Could the same thing be happening with clinicians who are willing to relax their advocacy duty for patients, but unwilling to take on the label of rationer?

Thinking Beyond the Individual Patient

Dr. Darren is about to perform a coronary arteriogram on Mr. Stevens and is deciding whether to use high-osmolar or low-osmolar contrast dye. He decides on the less expensive dye, even though he believes the more expensive one is less likely to cause complications. Dr. Darren reasons, "If everybody used the more expensive contrast dye, some patients would be better off, but not enough to justify the large increase in cost to society."

Dr. Darren has met all three criteria of bedside rationing. He has withheld the best contrast dye from the patient to save societal resources. Moreover, his justification (the benefits are "not enough to justify the large increase in cost to society") practically reads like part of the definition of bedside rationing. But that does not mean he acknowledges that he is rationing. Instead, by focusing on the *benefits* of his clinical decisions (it saves societal resources), Dr. Darren is able to overlook that he rationed from Mr. Stevens.

The tension between the cost of the alternative and its benefit is overt, but Dr. Darren displaces it from the single patient at hand to a wider field. He could have assumed an individual perspective and considered only the welfare of Mr. Stevens. Had he done so, he might have been uncomfortable choosing the less effective agent. Instead, he considers the effect across many other patients and many other clinicians.

Although consideration of society's financial interests is one of the three conditions of bedside rationing, clinicians may use it as a way of denying that they are rationing health care. In some practice settings, they are frequently reminded of the societal consequences of their clinical decisions. In county hospitals strapped for funds, most clinicians have seen examples of services that have been taken away from patients because of excessive spending in the previous fiscal year. When patients no longer have adequate access to social workers because of budget cuts, it makes clinicians think twice about ordering a marginally beneficial MRI. In such cases, it may be easy for them to characterize their actions as a good use of societal resources and not as bedside rationing. Indeed, some ethicists hold that bedside rationing is justifiable only in "closed systems," where savings will be guaranteed to go toward health care services for other patients (Daniels 1987). Whereas I propose that bedside rationing can be appropriate outside a closed system, clearly it is even more justifiable when the adverse consequences of pursuing marginally beneficial services are so direct.

Appealing to the Standard of Care

Mr. Green complains of a new, persistent headache. Dr. Brown orders a CT scan to evaluate the possibility of a brain tumor, even though she believes an MRI would be more likely to pick up a small tumor. In discussing the issue with Mr. Green, Dr. Brown mentions that, in general, a CT scan in this setting is the standard of care.

Dr. Brown opts against the more effective and more expensive MRI, suggesting to Mr. Green, or to herself, that the CT scan is the standard of care. Nevertheless, the standard of care is itself often influenced by considerations of societal cost. One reason it is not the standard of care to obtain MRIs in patients like Mr. Green is that the resulting costs would be high. If MRIs were less costly, the standard of care for patients with headache might be different.

It is possible to view Dr. Brown's actions many different ways. Is she playing with words to reduce social costs? Is she making peace with herself in a potentially difficult conflict? Is she following a long-standing professional norm that just happens to have internalized the consideration of social costs? Whatever the view, in many situations physicians appeal implicitly or explicitly to the standard of care; in many cases this implicitly reflects some consideration of cost; and yet most physicians in these situations probably do not feel that they are trading social cost for patient welfare.

In the survey of general internists discussed above, many respondents wrote about the importance of the standard of care in making these kinds of decisions. In the survey's vignettes, it cut both ways. Some physicians responded that it was appropriate to perform Pap smears every three years because that was the standard of care. Others wrote that yearly Pap smears are the standard of care. Some even remarked that the less effective screening strategy should be declared standard protocol by authorities, such as the American Cancer Society or the American Medical Association, so that physicians will have legal protection for withholding marginal benefits.

In any case, when the standard of care incorporates cost-worthiness judgments, as in this case or as in a recommendation for Pap smears every three years, clinicians may ration care without recognizing it. Because they are doing what everyone else does, in fact, what everyone else is *supposed* to do, and because rationing is impermissible, it is easy for them to think that, when they follow standard of care, they must not be rationing.

Changing the Standard of Evidence

During a visit with his internist Mr. Jones asks why he has not had a digital rectal examination in several years, the way he used to. Dr. Williams tells him that in the past the physicians in his practice routinely performed periodic rectal examinations because they believed it might detect prostate cancer and thereby save lives. Recently, Dr. Williams and his colleagues decided to abandon the practice after a review of the literature revealed no evidence that periodic digital rectal examination saves lives.

Dr. Williams's practice reversed an earlier decision and now advises against periodic screening with a digital rectal examination, a procedure that takes some time, has some equipment costs, and may induce other costs if abnormalities are detected. This reasoning embraces a positive standard of evidence similar to that of the U.S. Preventive Services Task Force (1996). But other standards might support more costly decisions. Organizations such as the American Cancer Society, for example, require a lower amount of evidence when evaluating cancer-screening technologies.

Is this new standard of evidence merely a convenient excuse to reduce costs? Or does it reflect a more rigorous approach to evaluating clinical practices? Proponents of evidence-based medicine would insist that the shift in the standard of evidence can be supported on independent grounds. Nevertheless, the rapid acceptance of this change almost certainly has something to do with its general concordance with cost containment.

Recent controversy about the appropriateness of mammography in women younger than fifty shows how value laden the standard of evidence can be. An expert panel was convened to review evidence about the efficacy of mammography in this group of women. The panel found no convincing evidence that mammography saves lives, although they were open to the possibility that such evidence was around the corner. They decided to make an agnostic recommendation (Fletcher 1997). They did not urge women to have the test or urge the medical community to withhold it. Instead, they decided it was a choice to be made by patients and their physicians. This agnostic recommendation, however, was greeted with outrage by those who believed that mammography ought to be made a routine part of medical practice for women under the age of fifty. The National Cancer Institute, which convened the panel, ignored the recommendation and came out in favor of routine mammography for women from age forty years. The standard of evidence required by the panel (some hard evidence of benefits from mammography in these women) was different from the standard of evidence acceptable to the National Cancer Institute and to many women's health advocates.

Displacing Blame

Ms. Lavedan sees her general internist, Dr. Mullaney, for the management of gastroesophageal reflux disease. When stomach acid is propelled backward up the esophagus, it causes significant heartburn and carries a long-term risk of esophageal cancer. Ms. Lavedan is surprised when Dr. Mullaney prescribes cimetidine rather than omeprazole, which she has heard so much about. Dr. Mullaney explains that although he believes omeprazole would probably be somewhat better at relieving Ms. Lavedan's symptoms, the health care company's formulary policy restricts its prescription to patients whose indication for the drug has been determined by a gastroenterologist.

Dr. Mullaney justifies or explains his less costly choice by appealing to an external rule. He apparently believes that one drug would be better than another, but displaces the blame for choosing the less effective, less expensive one onto someone else. The way one views this situation depends not only on clinical factors (for example, how much difference one perceives really exists between the agents), but also on professional and institutional factors (how much control Dr. Mullaney has in making a choice). Some of these rules may in fact be out of individual physicians' control, but others might not be. Perhaps the blame legitimately rests with the formulary committee. On the other hand, if Dr. Mullaney truly believes that omeprazole is better, he could refer Ms. Lavedan to a gastroenterologist.

Clinicians are facing increasing numbers of administrative hoops they must jump through before they can obtain beneficial services for patients. These hoops are put in place to control excessive spending by forcing clinicians to decide how many they will jump through to obtain specific services. Many times, administrators or third-party payers erect administrative barriers to direct clinicians away from marginally beneficial services. Clinicians may decide that a five-minute phone call is too high a price to pay to help a patient receive the best possible treatment when an adequate treatment can be obtained with less effort. In such cases, they are rationing at the bedside; they have relaxed their advocacy duties and decided that patients do not need specific services enough to justify the financial and opportunity costs of spending time to overcome administrative barriers.

Blame can be displaced, appropriately or not, in many different directions. The justification, "in general, we don't consider omeprazole first-line therapy for gastroesophageal reflux disease," in effect displaces responsibility for the decision from an individual physician to a professional norm. In doing so, it resembles the standard of care argument. Justifications such as "your policy doesn't cover a glucometer unless you require insulin" may reveal a firmer rule, although sometimes these can be bent. Physicians might blame the medical marketplace: "If I were to order an MRI for every patient with a headache I would be identified as a high-cost clinician, and managed care organizations would drop me from their panels." Or, they might displace responsibility to the patient: "Doxycycline is as effective an antibiotic as azithromycin; you simply have to take it longer." These justifications are similar in that they seek to displace the blame for perceived cost-quality tradeoffs away from the physician. In general, external rules are both limiting and liberating: a formulary decision that restricts access to expensive drugs can simultaneously tie physicians' hands and let them wash those hands of decisions they do not want to make.

Containing Costs Passively

The first time Ms. Lavedan came to Dr. Mullaney for the management of gastroesophageal reflux disease she requested a prescription for cimetidine because a friend of hers had a similar problem and received excellent relief with that agent. Dr. Mullaney believes omeprazole would be better at relieving Ms. Lavedan's symptoms, but thinks that its higher cost precludes prescribing it as a first-line agent. He, thus, happily agrees with Ms. Lavedan and writes a prescription for cimetidine.

Although this case is similar to the previous one, here Dr. Mullaney is spared the need to provide an explanation for his choice of the less expensive, less effective agent. It was certainly convenient for him that Ms. Lavedan expressed her preferences the way she did.

One way to view this situation is to recognize that patient preferences should always be considered when making medical choices. Patient preferences for medical rather than surgical approaches to certain conditions may reflect deep attitudes about risk or aggressiveness (Singer et al. 1991). But incorporating expressed preferences into medical decision making may be insufficient if patients' understanding of available alternatives is inadequate. Ms. Lavedan may not have heard of omeprazole, and Dr. Mullaney did not give her his impression of that drug's superiority. Although he did exactly what Ms. Lavedan requested, he took a passive stance in serving as her advocate.

Making do with Less than the Best

Mrs. Glenn sees her family practitioner, Dr. Shepard, for referral to an orthopedist for total knee replacement. There are two orthopedists in the community. Dr. Aldrin is considered a national expert in the procedure, but the plan under which Dr. Shepard sees Mrs. Glenn has an arrangement with Dr. Grissom, a general orthopedist. Dr. Shepard anticipates Mrs. Glenn's concern: "I know that you would like a referral to Dr. Aldrin because she is considered the expert at knee replacements, but Dr. Grissom is an able orthopedist."

One can imagine many different financial or organizational reasons why Dr. Shepard refers Mrs. Glenn to Dr. Grissom, and they might affect how one views the situation. Common to any of these unstated arrangements is whether Dr. Shepard's responsibility is to arrange the best possible care for Mrs. Glenn or simply good care. Even if Dr. Aldrin really is the best, perhaps she could not possibly operate on all of the patients in the community. Such immutable constraints increase our tolerance for making do, and might make Dr. Shepard more comfortable with his actions even if he would have referred his mother to Dr. Aldrin.

Many general internists responding to our survey explained their responses with language that echoed this alternative characterization of rationing. One wrote: "A 90% effective test is really very good at screening. You wouldn't be missing much." Another wrote: "This does not seem to be rationing but, instead, merely distributing sufficient care in a cost-effective manner." And another: "Given alternative choices for diagnosis and treatment with little or no statistical difference in outcome, one should certainly pursue the less expensive route."

Giving the Best Treatment only after Others Fail

Ms. Corell's general internist, Dr. Greeno, is managing her high cholesterol. He thinks it is reasonable to try a less expensive cholesterol-lowering drug first, and graduate to a more expensive one only if the first one does not adequately reduce her cholesterol even though Mrs. Corell's insurance would cover the added cost of the more expensive agent.

It takes a broad definition of "compromise" to state that Dr. Greeno is compromising Ms. Corell's care to save some money. After all, he intends to prescribe the expensive agent that he believes is more effective—but only if the less expensive one fails. Many times physicians start with an inexpensive approach and move to a more costly and more effective one if necessary.

We might think differently if Dr. Greeno used to prescribe the more expensive drug as first-line therapy in similar cases, but developed this new strategy only after his health care company introduced financial incentives favoring the less expensive drug. Still, some maintain that he should have been following a strategy like this all along. Nevertheless, if he really believes that one drug is more likely to succeed than the other, he has made a (small) compromise in the care of Ms. Corell: he withheld the most beneficial service to save money. If money had been irrelevant, he would clearly have chosen the more expensive drug. He rationed from Ms. Corell.

Alternative Characterizations and Bedside Rationing

Bedside rationing is pervasive, varied, and often disguised. Sometimes clinicians ration from their patients but use hidden language to describe the situation. Often that language provides a justification for rationing without admitting that it is rationing. As physicians, patients, insurers, and others face trade-offs between cost and quality, the debate should not be about some global notion of rationing or compromise, but about which justifications are valid and which compromises are appropriate.

Given the ubiquity of bedside rationing, by whatever name it goes by, it is time to see whether any moral arguments can justify the practice and, if so, find out what that means about the appropriateness of using CEA to guide these decisions.

9

The Unbearable Rightness of Bedside Rationing

In chapter 6 I exposed bedside rationing's unseemly underbelly: it violates clinicians' advocacy duties, thereby threatening the trust necessary for a good clinician-patient relationship. Moreover, clinicians untrained in how to ration will do so in a discriminatory manner and in ways that may not even provide savings that go toward improved patient care. In chapter 8 I argued that bedside rationing is ubiquitous, that many clinicians approve of actions that qualify as bedside rationing, and that many clinicians find enough euphemisms for it to convince themselves that they are not personally involved in such practices.

Are clinicians fooling themselves or their patients by using euphemisms to cover up immoral rationing activities?

Clearly, they are using euphemisms to avoid having to admit to themselves or others what they are doing. Euphemisms exist to make uncomfortable truths easier to swallow. But in this case they do not exist primarily to hide immoral activities. Instead, they enable clinicians to conduct *appropriate* bedside rationing.

"Appropriate bedside rationing?" you say. "That's an oxymoron! What about trust, advocacy, fiduciary duty, and discriminatory rationing?"

These are very good questions. My short answer to them is this: although bedside rationing is morally problematic, these problems have been exaggerated, and no acceptable rationing plan will succeed at containing health care costs without some amount of it. Yet, in the current health care environment, most clinicians have been taught that it is immoral. Thus, they rely on euphemisms, often appropriately, without having to acknowledge that they are rationing.

My long answer to this question is . . . this chapter. Here I contend that bedside rationing can be a morally acceptable part of medical practice. In arguing for its (occasional) moral appropriateness, I walk down two rhetorical roads. First, I challenge the moral inappropriateness of bedside rationing. I revisit the main moral criticisms presented in chapter 6 and propose that many of them have been overstated. Second, I maintain that bedside rationing is unavoidable if we want to control health care costs in an acceptable manner. No acceptable alternative mechanism will succeed without relying, in part, on bedside rationing.

Revisiting the Supposed Evilness of Bedside Rationing

Revisiting Clinicians' Advocacy Duties

Lawyers and physicians advocate for clients and patients because they have important knowledge to help them through significant events. But the analogy between the professionals is far from perfect (Hall 1997). Lawyers are required to be absolute advocates for clients because the legal system is adversarial. They fight for clients' best interests because someone else's lawyers are doing the opposite. If one group of lawyers puts forth less than 100% effort, the outcome of its legal cases will not be fair. No such adversarial system exists in medicine. Thus, physicians' advocacy duties are less absolute than lawyers'.

Some wonder whether the growth of managed care makes the analogy between lawyers and physicians stronger. Managed care organizations, by this view, fight against patients' best interests while clinicians advocate for them. But this view is a distortion. It is unfair to accuse all managed care organizations of explicitly engaging in such a fight. Moreover, the last thing we should want is a health care system that resembles the adversarial nature of the legal system. Instead, we should strive for a system in which third-party payers and clinicians work together to promote patients' interests within a context of resource constraints. Indeed, if clinicians insist on pursuing patients' best interests without regard to costs, we will inevitably end up with an adversarial system in which patients and clinicians face increasing obstacles to good health care while third-party payers construct ever more elaborate and burdensome administrative rationing mechanisms.

Clinicians have important advocacy duties for their patients, but these duties are not absolute. Certainly, as third-party payers increase their efforts to withhold appropriate care from patients, clinicians must increase their advocacy. But when, in the name of societal resource management, third-party payers try to decrease the use of marginally beneficial services, clinicians should not always assume that their moral duty is to circumvent these efforts. They must decide which battles to fight for their patients, and they must decide when it is acceptable to allow third-party payers to restrict patients' access to beneficial services.

Revisiting Patients' Trust in Clinicians

The American media are abuzz with stories of managed care companies withholding care from patients. In some of these stories, physicians are seen as patient advocates, busy fighting the system, but in others they are seen as partners in crime. Similarly, primary care clinicians tell stories of patients questioning their motives for avoiding unnecessary radiographs or for recommending that patients allow themselves a chance to recover spontaneously from an illness before launching a diagnostic work-up. These anecdotes suggest that patients are worried about physicians' complicity in widespread efforts to control health care costs.

However, these anecdotes hardly pass as evidence that bedside rationing has reduced people's trust in clinicians. Indeed, counteranecdotes abound. Fee-for-service ophthalmologists, for example, have been questioned by patients about whether the physicians' recommendations for cataract operations are influenced by their mortgage payments. Traditional fee-for-service systems have always had the potential to decrease patients' trust in clinicians. Nevertheless, physicians remain one of the most highly trusted professional groups, despite evidence that many of them have abused the fee-for-service system to advance their financial interests. As most countries depart from this traditional system into ones that emphasize cost containment, some physicians could once again find ways to promote their financial gain rather than promote patients' best interests. But these abuses may or may not significantly affect patients' trust. Although we ought to be concerned about how bedside rationing affects clinician-patient relationships, it is far too early to conclude that trimming marginal benefits from patients will damage these relationships.

Early evidence suggests that, rather than lose trust in clinicians who ration at the bedside, people might even approve of the practice. In a survey of Minnesotans, most respondents said that if health care has to be rationed, they prefer that physicians decide how to do it rather than legislators or health care administrators (Miles & Bendiksen 1994). This response should be interpreted cautiously. Rather than endorsing bedside rationing, these Minnesotans may have been endorsing physicians' roles in other types of rationing, such as through formulary committees. In addition, people may approve of bedside rationing in theory but disapprove of it when visiting their primary care clinicians. Despite these cautions, the survey should remind us that we do not yet know whether or how much bedside rationing will erode patients' trust in clinicians. Clearly we need more research in this area.

Until we know more about this, we must make a judgment call. We must decide how much of the clinician-patient relationship we will risk damaging to contain health care costs. Some may think no risk should be accepted. But this view ignores the risks we have already accepted by having a fee-for-service system. In fact, even salary-based systems carry risks; patients may wonder, for example, whether recommendations to delay surgery are based on medical reasoning or professional laziness. Any system of incentives, whether it encourages physicians to do more, to do less, or to do nothing, could potentially damage the relationship.

In making a judgment call regarding how much bedside rationing will damage these relationships, we must consider the likelihood that patients will be unaware that clinicians are rationing from them. In many, probably most, cases patients will have no idea that a benefit is being withheld. As I stated, bedside rationing is ubiquitous, but is often invisible even to the clinicians doing it. If *physicians* are often unaware that they are rationing care, as suggested by the survey of general internists discussed in the previous chapter, patients are unlikely to be aware.

For example, the VA hospital where I practice has a mild shortage of gastroenterologists. We have enough to take care of patients' urgent and semiurgent gastroenterological needs, but not enough to justify referrals for routine matters. The situation is similar to that facing many managed care systems, where specialists are a scarce commodity who must be used carefully. In my case, I am less likely to refer patients to the gastro-enterology clinic.

Is my hesitancy an example of bedside rationing? Yes. At times a referral offers a small probability of benefit and, without resource constraints, I would refer patients to a gastroenterologist. But, because it would add to other patients' waiting times, I choose not to refer patients; I think the small chance of them benefiting is not worth the additional strain on limited gastroenterological resources, and does not justify any increase in additional waiting time for other (typically needier) patients.

My occasional hesitancy in this regard is an example of bedside rationing. But how often are my patients aware that I have rationed? Literally hundreds of times a month most primary care physicians could refer patients to subspecialists, but choose not to because they think the visit is only marginally beneficial. Patients with chest pain are not immediately referred to cardiologists because primary care clinicians can treat them effectively; yet in a world without resource constraints, primary care clinicians would increase their requests to cardiologists to evaluate these patients. Most patients are probably unaware of these instances.

Consider the invisibility of rationing colon cancer screening. There are many ways to screen for colon cancer, mainly, fecal occult blood testing, colonoscopy, flexible sigmoidoscopy, and barium enema. The most effective test to decrease colon cancer deaths is colonoscopy, but it is expensive, labor intensive, and painful. Thus, it is rarely recommended as the screening test of choice. Instead, clinicians screen patients with some combination of flexible sigmoidoscopy and fecal occult blood testing, the two least accurate and least expensive tests.

If money were irrelevant, colonoscopy would be performed increasingly. Although it is uncomfortable and poses some risks, it allows gastroenterologists to visualize the entire colon and to remove any abnormal tissue at the time, thus both diagnosing and treating at the same time. If money were irrelevant, the frequency of colon cancer screening, by whatever methods, would increase. Rather than examine people every seven or ten years, clinicians would screen them every five years or every three years, much as they would increase Pap smear screening from every three years to every year. If money were irrelevant, clinicians would be more likely to order radiographs that visualize the entire colon rather than rely on flexible sigmoidoscopies, which visualize only the last 60 centimeters. But money is not irrelevant. Radiographs and colonoscopy prevent colon cancer at significant costs—hundreds of thousands of dollars per cancer detected. Money is influencing these decisions and patients have little idea of the fact.

Screening decisions are inevitably decisions about cost-effectiveness (Eddy et al. 1987). For most diseases, the public does not have strong attitudes about how or how often they want to be screened. Clinicians' decisions are accepted without any suspicions that cost-worthiness judgments have been made. (Breast and prostate cancer screening are notable exceptions. Debates about whether to screen women age 40 years with mammography or elderly men with PSA test have entered into public consciousness in ways atypical for most screening tests.) For example, few people worry about whether they have been screened for thyroid disease; and how many complain that their physicians forgot to screen them for parathyroid disease with a serum calcium test?

Some will object at this point that, if bedside rationing is ubiquitous, and if patients do not know about it, physicians are being immorally incommunicative. Patients, they will insist, deserve to know about clinicians' rationing decisions (Levinsky 1998).

But this objection ignores the practical reality of the typical doctor-patient encounter. Even during a routine examination, there are an enormous number of important things to discuss. Does the patient wear a seat belt in the car? Is there a loaded gun at home? Is the patient a victim of domestic violence? Is the patient suffering chest pain, urinary frequency, diarrhea, weight loss . . . ? In addition, clinicians have to give patients a chance to talk about symptoms that are plaguing them. Finally, clinicians must teach patients about their illnesses, talk to them about how often to take pills, and show them how to use equipment such as inhalers. This huge agenda, often crammed into a fifteen- or twenty-minute time slot, forces clinicians to set priorities. For example, many screen for domestic violence only in high-risk patients, if at all. That means some cases of domestic violence are undetected. Given this huge agenda, how important is it to tell patients that they could have had their thyroid-stimulating hormone or a calcium level measured, or that they could have undergone colon cancer screening every three years instead of every seven years? How important is it to mention that, in a perfect world, a dermatologist would have glanced at their rash rather than having them try a steroid cream prescribed by their family physician?

Whereas it is possible to improve communication between clinicians and patients, it would be a poor use of time for clinicians to discuss every small health care benefit they chose not to pursue. They have more valuable things to do with their time than discuss every marginally beneficial service that they withheld. For these reasons, it is unlikely that patients will be aware of most bedside rationing and, therefore, unlikely that it will erode their trust in clinicians.

Revisiting Whether Clinicians Are Trained to Ration Health Care

Opponents of bedside rationing are correct to say that clinicians have not been trained in the techniques and that, in part because of this lack, they are prone to ration in ways that are haphazard or, worse yet, discriminatory. This is an important reason for clinicians to be very cautious about how and when they ration at the bedside. This is also the reason why we must teach them to interpret CEA, so that their rationing decisions can be guided by some of its central insights.

But lack of formal training is not a persuasive reason to forbid physicians from rationing. To begin with, they are not the only people who have no training in this area. I do not know *anyone* who has really been trained in how to ration health care. Business schools, health care administration schools, and public policy schools do not educate students how to do it. Legislators are certainly not trained in these matters. And whereas philosophers and ethicists understand moral theories of justice, they do not have practical training in how to make real-world rationing decisions.

Despite lack of formal training, physicians have more experience in health care rationing than any other professionals. As we have seen, physicians have been taught to think about the public health consequences of how they prescribe antibiotics (Lipsitch 1995). They are frequently reminded that broad-spectrum antibiotics should be reserved for cases of serious, life-threatening infections, or for infections with pathogens known to be resistant to less broad-spectrum agents. Pressure to withhold the drugs occurs to minimize the development of antibiotic resistance. In many cases this means physicians withhold the best treatment from a patient to decrease the long-term risks to society at large. Similarly, physicians have always rationed the amount of time they spend with patients. Time pressures have grown in recent years, but even when routine visits were thirty minutes instead of fifteen, as they are today, physicians had to set priorities. They had to decide which issues were most important to deal with during those thirty minutes.

Just because clinicians are experienced with rationing, of course, does not mean that they know how to ration ethically, but at least they are familiar with the trade-offs involved in making these decisions. Indeed, they do many things routinely that they are not formally trained to do. I never had a nutrition course in medical school (a common oversight that most medical schools have now corrected), but I have learned something about nutrition and can talk about it intelligently with my patients. Much of what physicians learn about caring for patients is learned through experience, as are many of their rationing practices. They are taught to ration by seeing how more experienced clinicians do it, and by being encouraged to see another patient every fifteen minutes.

Clearly, physicians need more formal training about how to ration health care. But right now, they and other clinicians probably have more experience with the procedures than any other health care professionals.

Revisiting Whether Bedside Rationing Violates Patients' Best Interests
Earlier I discussed how health insurance, like a single restaurant check, increases the demand for health care services. This places physicians in a moral dilemma. Imagine a group of people each of whom is at a 1/10,000 risk of developing a painful disease. A new, $100 blood test is available to detect this disease, so it can be treated. No patient thinks the test is worth $100, but Mr. Thrifty asks his physician for it, reasoning that he will only have to pay a $5 copayment. This leaves his physician in a dilemma. At a cost of $1 million per disease detected, the test is not very cost effective. But the patient shielded from most of these costs, wants the test. What is the right thing to do?

Opponents of bedside rationing would examine the moral implications of this decision from the viewpoint of the individual patient, from which the choice seems clear. The test will benefit Thrifty at a small cost to him.

Because it is in Thrifty's best interest to spend $5 on the test, his physician has a moral obligation to order it.

But this ignores the importance of thinking about the consequences of generalizing particular behaviors (Singer 1971). Suppose every physician concludes that bedside rationing is wrong and therefore honors the requests of their patients to receive the test. As a result, all patients would pay $100 to receive the blood test (by means of increased insurance premiums) even though none would think it was worth the money. This seems absurd. By collectively pursuing individual patients' best interests, physicians leave all patients with less money and more medical care than they want. Other examples raise their own problems. If Thrifty's physician is the only one to conclude that bedside rationing is wrong, and thus is the only one to order the blood test, his patient will pay $5 for the blood test and the rest of the cost will be picked up by all the other patients. Thrifty, in effect, will be a free rider, obtaining all the benefit while others pay most of the cost. Alternatively, the physician could decide not to order the blood test for Thrifty while everyone else's physician did order it. The consequence would be that Thrifty would contribute almost $100 to the pot without having the test himself.

The physician's dilemma is this: no matter what other physicians do, his own patients will always benefit by having the blood test. However, the collective consequence of pursuing each patient's individual interests is that all patients have the blood test and all pay $100, and therefore everyone is worse off.

It is not in patients' best collective interests to purchase marginally beneficial health care services simply because their cost is subsidized by health insurance. I am not trying to say that health insurance causes all medical services to be a waste of money. Indeed, this is an extreme example used to illustrate my point and is not representative of the types of services offered to most patients. But rationing such marginally beneficial services would not necessarily violate patients' best interests if we interpret those interests broadly.

Revisiting Whether Bedside Rationing Is Appropriate Only When Savings Go Toward Other Health Care Services

Usually, when physicians save money by withholding marginally beneficial services, they cannot be sure how this saved money will be spent. There is no guarantee, for example, that it will be used to provide other, more beneficial health services to other patients.

But why should we require that savings from bedside rationing must go to purchase other health care services? When physicians ration at the bedside, they should be thinking about patients' interests in the broadest sense. If specific health care services are not worth their cost, clinicians ought to withhold them regardless of what the savings are used for. We take too narrow a view of justice when we forbid physicians from rationing marginally beneficial services, at the same time that many of our governments cannot figure out how to pay exponentially rising health care bills, when small businesses in the United States cannot afford health insurance for their employees, and when large businesses struggle to compete with foreign companies that have lower medical costs. Government employers and consumers are sending a strong message that we are spending too much money on health care. Consequently, sometimes it is appropriate to spend money saved by bedside rationing to purchase nonhealth care goods.

This raises another question. Should money saved by health care rationing be required to go toward other social welfare goods? Must physicians have proof that the money saved on thyroid screening tests, for example, will go toward education for underserved populations, crime prevention, or some other laudable social goal? Whereas it would be nice to put more money into these important programs, people have lots of ideas about where they want to spend their money. Sometimes people think buying a new VCR would be more beneficial than having a thyroid screening test. When physicians withhold marginally beneficial services they free up money that could reduce government debt, increase insurance company revenues, or fatten patients' wallets. If the test is not worth its expense, chances are the money will be better spent elsewhere.

The Moral Strengths of Bedside Rationing

So far I have insisted that many of the moral problems associated with bedside rationing are overstated. If this were my only argument in support of bedside rationing, it would be unconvincing. Even if bedside rationing is only a little evil rather than a very large one, it would still require moral justification. For it to be morally acceptable, its moral strengths must, at least in some circumstances, outweigh its moral weaknesses. What are its moral strengths?

Bedside rationing has two moral strengths. First, it is indispensable. If we hope to reduce the use of extremely costly health care services that bring tiny health benefits, society should not be spending $1 million to produce one QALY. But, as I propose, it will be very difficult to eliminate these services without the help of bedside rationing. Second, bedside rationing allows our health care to be rationed in ways that account for patients' individual characteristics. In contrast, broad rationing rules must necessarily make decisions about how to deal with the average patient. Let me elaborate on both of these moral strengths.

No Acceptable Rationing Mechanism Can Succeed at Controlling Health Care Costs without the Help of Bedside Rationing

Imagine a formulary committee that is trying to reduce the cost of ulcer therapy for its health system. Physicians in the health system have increasingly been prescribing proton pump inhibitors, an expensive class of drugs that cure ulcers more effectively than less expensive ones such as cimetidine. The formulary committee decides that from now on, physicians will be required to treat patients' ulcers with cimetidine or some other less expensive alternative rather than proton pump inhibitors.

Now imagine a physician who is hell-bent on pursuing her patient's best interests and will look for a way to provide proton pump inhibitors for them. How will she do this? Perhaps the formulary committee allows proton pump inhibitors to be prescribed for the treatment of reflux disease, which is closely related to ulcers. The physician could interpret the patient's symptoms as being suggestive of reflux disease. (In fact, the symptoms of reflux disease and ulcer disease are often hard to distinguish without further investigation, such as a stomach film.) She could prescribe proton pump inhibitors regardless of whether patients have ulcer disease or reflux, thereby circumventing the formulary committee restriction.

This physician's extensive prescription of proton pump inhibitors might force the formulary committee to find a way to prevent physicians from reclassifying patients with ulcers as having reflux. Perhaps the committee requires physicians to perform stomach radiographs or endoscopy to confirm the diagnosis of reflux disease before allowing them to prescribe these drugs. But that would be expensive (radiographs and endoscopies are not cheap), and it would require the committee to monitor performance of the tests. Perhaps, instead, the committee simply forbids primary care physicians from prescribing proton pump inhibitors and allows only gastroenterologists this privilege. This, too, has resource implications. Primary care physicians advocating for patients' best interests would be compelled to refer all patients with ulcers to gastroenterologists.

Imagine, instead of such burdensome formulary committee rules, administrators in the health system decide to make it so difficult for physicians to obtain specific drugs, such as proton pump inhibitors, that the physicians will throw up their hands and prescribe less expensive and slightly less effective agents. Perhaps the health system requires clinicians to fill out an extra form to prescribe expensive drugs. Maybe it orders physicians to call subspecialists for approval to write such prescriptions. None of these obstacles would get in the way of clinicians dedicated to pursuing patients' best interests.

Imagine a patient in an examination room with her primary care physician. If this patient's best interests were all that mattered to this physician, he would make any phone calls and fill out any forms necessary to promote her best interests. Indeed, if administrative obstacles to providing the best possible health care were rare, an occasional five-minute phone call or an occasional ten minutes spent filling out paperwork would not be a significant burden. But as pressures to contain costs have grown, these administrative hurdles have become common. For any single patient, it sounds relatively easy to spend an extra five or ten minutes to make sure he or she will receive the best available drug rather than the second best. Multiplying this type of five- or ten-minute investment by every other patient a clinician sees in a day makes it impossible to pursue each one's best interests. At some point, clinicians have to give patients less than the best, rather than spend the time it takes to break through administrative barriers.

If clinicians spent fifteen minutes with each patient pursuing a marginally beneficial service that could be obtained only through this extra effort, they would have difficulty taking care of all their other patients, or of getting home at night to see their families. This reveals that clinicians must relax their advocacy duties so that they can take care of more important problems, such as the next patient waiting. They must allow patients to go with less than the best, even though it is within their power, for specific patients, to provide the best possible medical care.

Rationing Mechanisms that Do Not Involve Bedside Rationing Are Too Imprecise to Ration Appropriately

If physicians want to pursue patients' best interests, they will find ways to do so. Keeping them from doing so will succeed only with complex and burdensome rules limiting their behavior (Mechanic 1992), and even then success is not guaranteed. Clearly we must have rules to keep physicians from spending too much money, and physicians are going to have to get used to the idea that their clinical decisions will be increasingly monitored and regulated. But some of this ridiculously complex rule making would be unnecessary if physicians simply agreed, on occasion, to do less than the best for their patients. If they decided that a course of cimetidine was a reasonable way to start treating most patients with ulcer disease, the health system might not have to make burdensome rules governing use of proton pump inhibitors, stomach films, or gastrointestinal referrals.

Most theories of justice insist that like people should be treated alike. But global rationing rules are often unable to distinguish which patients are alike in clinically (and morally) relevant ways. In Oregon's Medicaid rationing plan, after it abandoned cost-effectiveness, the final list of services determined that the state would no longer reimburse physicians for treating Medicaid patients with sarcoidosis, an inflammatory condition that remits spontaneously in most people.

This decision in no way implies that medical treatment of people with sarcoidosis *never* brings substantial benefits, or that physicians could not identify such patients. In fact, some patients gain great benefit from treatment. Nevertheless, Oregon could not fit such subtleties into its list of covered and uncovered services. Instead, it had to make a global decision about which ones to pay for, even if that meant cutting out some people who could gain from treatment. In no way do I mean this as a criticism of Oregon. I do not know of any more thorough and better-intended effort to ration health care than theirs. But, rationing from the top down inevitably forces patients and clinicians to fit into a relatively small number of prespecified categories. Top-down rationing that does not rely on physicians to decide when to ration health care, but that ties physicians' hands to take the burden away from them, necessarily relies on imprecise rules that may not fit the specific circumstances any patient faces. The downside of rationing health care solely according to administrative rules is that it is necessarily imprecise and directs its blows across large swaths of patients, whereas physicians rationing at the bedside could more easily determine which patients would or would not benefit from treatment.

The Unbearable Rightness of Bedside Rationing

Bedside rationing raises a number of important moral concerns. But without it, without some relaxation of clinicians' traditional duties to advocate for patients' best interests, it is difficult to imagine an acceptable and feasible way of containing health care costs. Fortunately, the associated moral problems (many of which have been overstated) can be minimized if clinicians' bedside rationing activities are limited to reducing marginally beneficial services that bring small or infrequent benefits at great financial cost. It is nearly impossible to get worked up about a physician who decides not to order thyroid screening tests for young male patients, who rarely (very rarely) develop thyroid disease. And it is difficult to imagine patients loosing trust when clinicians schedule follow-up visits at four-month rather than three-month intervals.

If clinicians do not ration at the bedside, third-party payers will be forced to tie clinicians' hands. They will restrict clinicians from using specific services or punish them for using too many resources. Returning to the proton pump inhibitor example, clinicians have a choice. If they resist efforts to reduce proton pump inhibitor use, third-party payers will forbid *all* use of the agents or will find ways (painfully bureaucratic ways, no doubt) to ensure that the drugs are prescribed only for specific types of patients. In contrast, if clinicians recognize third-party payer attempts to reduce proton pump inhibitor use as a sign that society wants to decrease health care costs, clinicians will accept the restrictions and order these drugs only after trying less expensive ones, and try to circumvent the rules only for patients with specific needs that are not captured by the rationing guideline.

Cost-effectiveness analysis offers the type of information that could guide these decisions. It can help identify health care interventions that bring small or rare benefits at great financial cost. In addition, it can formalize clinicians' thinking about rationing. If clinicians relied solely on cost-effectiveness to guide their rationing decisions, they would be unlikely to ration haphazardly or discriminatorily. Moreover, they would potentially be able to identify patients for whom the cost-effectiveness of an intervention was not well captured by CEA.

I do not by any means think that clinicians should ration solely according to cost-effectiveness. Throughout this book I have pointed out a number of problems with the ways CEA sets health care priorities. These problems preclude CEA as the sole way for anyone, including clinicians at the bedside, to ration health care. Nevertheless, as I discuss in more detail in chapter 11, clinicians may be able to use CEA to guide their rationing decisions while considering other factors. In other words, they may be able to take advantage of the strengths of CEA while minimizing its weaknesses.

Certainly CEA is an imperfect rationing tool, and bedside rationing is a flawed mechanism. But as Winston Churchill said about democracy, in many instances, the alternatives to rationing at the bedside according, in part, to CEA are even worse. Rationing is a messy business. We should be suspicious of anyone who thinks a single mechanism will solve all of the related dilemmas. For now, clinicians have to relax their advocacy duties to help minimize the use of health care interventions that bring small or rare benefits at a great cumulative financial cost. In the future, we can hope to improve the way we identify these interventions and improve the way clinicians use this information to guide their rationing decisions.

III

The Future of Cost-Effectiveness Analysis
and Health Care Rationing

10

Future Possibilities for Improving How Cost-Effectiveness Analysis Incorporates Public Rationing Preferences

Dr. Armstrong works in a large multispecialty practice that has contracted with most of the local managed care organizations. Business is booming, but dollars are tight because the two largest managed care organizations in town dominate the local marketplace and have negotiated exceedingly low reimbursement rates with the group. Dr. Armstrong is well paid, but his salary has not risen for two years. More important, his group is facing tough times. There is even some discussion of laying off employees.

Dr. Armstrong and his colleagues have worked hard to eliminate wasteful medical practices. But further cost containment will, by necessity, come at the expense of patient care. It is time, Dr. Armstrong admits to himself, to stop doing everything possible to benefit his patients. Some benefits are simply too expensive. They are not worth their price. And they are certainly not sufficiently worth while to send some of his close friends to the unemployment line.

Where should Dr. Armstrong turn to identify which services to ration? What can the multispecialty group do to keep from going bankrupt and still offer high-quality medical care to its patients?

There is no simple way for Dr. Armstrong and his colleagues to answer these questions. These questions will probably never have simple answers. But in the future, it is possible for CEA to give these physicians a much better way of making difficult rationing decisions. To do this, however, CEA has to be improved.

Earlier in this book I presented data showing that CEA does not ration health care the way many people would want it done. At the same time, I showed that many people's preferences are difficult to interpret and are sometimes so inconsistent that it is difficult to imagine how they could be translated into sensible policies.

Although it is extremely difficult to capture public rationing preferences, a more modest goal may be attainable: to determine values that deserve to be incorporated into CEA so it captures the public's approximate preferences better. Most experts do not think that utility measurement perfectly captures the quality of life of various health conditions, and most do not think it perfectly places health states on an interval scale. Nevertheless, utility measurement comes closer to capturing the quality of life of various health states than would a system that ignored the process altogether. Even if no such thing as a perfect measure of health-related quality of life exists, few deny the importance of trying to measure quality of life. Similarly, no true measure of people's rationing preferences may be available, but we ought to do what we can to make sure that CEA measurements come closer to these preferences than they do currently.

In previous chapters I discussed three values held by many members of the general public that are not currently accounted for in CEA: people want to give priority to severely ill patients, even when their treatment is not very cost effective; people want to give greater priority to life-saving treatments in people with chronic illness and disability than would be given to them in a QALY-based rationing system; and people want health care services or health care outcomes to be distributed fairly, even if this lowers the average health of the population. If we decided ("we" being either society at large or health care experts or some other decision-making group) that these three values deserve to play a role in policy decisions, would that require us to abandon CEA as a priority-setting tool? Or could CEA be modified to incorporate some or all of these values?

In this chapter I propose that CEA is flexible enough to accommodate a wide range of values in its measurements. Indeed, QALYs themselves are a relatively recent improvement, and allow CEA to accommodate values for improving quality of life rather than accounting only for how health care interventions affect the length of people's lives. In the spirit of QALY measurement, other values can also be incorporated into CEA. To show this, I briefly review how it mathematically incorporates QALY measurement and time-discounting measurement into its mathematical framework. This will help demonstrate its mathematical flexibility. Then I show which of these three values could potentially be mathematically incorporated into CEA. Ultimately, I suggest that CEA can accommodate more values than it currently does, although public preferences for distributing health care resources fairly may never be quantifiable in ways useful for CEA. In other words, CEA measurement can and should be improved, but it will still be an imperfect moral guide for rationing health care.

Values Currently Incorporated into CEA

As we have seen, the measurement of cost-effectiveness is, by its nature, one of value (Williams 1992). Most obviously, it looks at the dollar value of the costs of medical interventions, but it also takes account of other values. Through QALY measurement, it places value on health care treatments that do not necessarily lengthen life but improve the quality of life. In addition, through time discounting, CEA places greater value on interventions that produce health benefits immediately versus ones that produce benefits in the future.

Placing Value on Quality of Life

As I have explained, CEA incorporates utilities into its measurements to show how money can be spent in ways that maximize the improvement in people's health-related utility, or health-related quality of life. This is an explicit acknowledgment that most people think the goal of health care should not only be to save or prolong lives, but also to improve people's health-related quality of life. Before the introduction of QALYs, CEAs primarily reported the number of dollars it took for an intervention to save a life or to produce an additional year of life. It paid no attention to quality of life. Without QALYs, it was impossible to compare the relative cost-effectiveness of life-prolonging versus life-improving interventions, much less interventions that did both. Through QALY measurement, CEA places greater value on treatments that produce full health than on treatments that produce less than full health.

It is important to understand how CEA *mathematically* incorporates utility values into its measurements, so that its flexibility to incorporate other values will be clear. In CEA, the duration of benefit brought by a health care intervention is multiplied by the improvement in quality of life (or utility) brought by the intervention. If an intervention adds three years to someone's life at a utility of 0.5, it adds:

3 years × 0.5 utility gain = 1.5 QALYs.

If an intervention adds three years of perfect health in half of patients and three years at a utility of 0.5 in the other half, it produces:

(3 years × 1 utility gain × 0.5 probability) + (3 years × 0.5 utility gain × 0.5 probability) = 2.25 QALYs.

Placing Value on Receiving Health Benefits Now Rather than Later

Imagine two interventions. The first will bring immediate health benefits to several patients, thereby producing 1.5 QALYs over the next two years. The second will benefit three patients and produce 1.5 QALYs, but these patients will not receive the benefits for ten years. If maximizing QALYs was the sole goal of health care spending, these two interventions would be equally important. However, many people think that interventions that bring benefits now ought to be given more priority than those that produce benefits later.

In addition to incorporating people's preferences for improving quality of life, CEA incorporates preferences for receiving health care benefits that occur now rather than later. To do this, it *discounts* future benefits so that they are worth less than current benefits (Gold et al. 1996; Krahn & Gafni 1993; Olsen 1993). The easiest way to understand the reason for discounting future benefits is to think about most people's attitudes toward money. Most people would rather have $100 given to them now than have $100 given to them one year from now. This is so, in part, because people favor present consumption over future consumption. (How else can we justify buying an expensive hardcover book when we know the paperback will be out in twelve months?) It is also true because $100 invested now will usually be worth more than $100 a year from now. This preference can be captured by discounting future money. For example, a discount rate of 3% reflects a view that receiving $100 now is equivalent to receiving $103 a year from now.

Health benefits can be discounted in the same way as monetary benefits, although there is more debate about how best to measure such preferences (Gold et al. 1996; Weinstein 1986). In current CEA models, a year of healthy life gained in the future will be discounted at a rate of 3% to 5% per year. For example, imagine two health care programs, one of which will prevent life-threatening illness in a population, thereby producing 100 additional years of healthy life. The other intervention cures people of a life-threatening illness and, for the same cost, also produces 100 extra years of healthy life. These two interventions produce the same health benefits. However, if the preventive intervention does not produce benefits for many years, CEA would discount those benefits and the curative intervention would be seen as more cost effective and thus deserving greater priority.

The appropriate discount rate for health benefits is hotly debated (Krahn & Gafni 1993; Olsen 1993; Redelmeier & Heller 1993). Controversy also surrounds whether people truly discount health benefits the same way they discount future monetary gains. The key point for this discussion, however, is not whether CEA accurately captures public attitudes toward the discounting of future health benefits. Instead, it focuses on discounting to show how CEA is able to accommodate values into its mathematical framework.

A Mathematical Illustration of How CEA Incorporates Preferences to Improve Quality of Life and to Receive Benefits Now Rather than Later

Quality of life measurement and time discounting are used to adjust the value of life years gained in CEAs. To illustrate these adjustments, figure 10.1 shows the result of a CEA for an intervention that extends a patient's life for one year in a suboptimal state of health (with a utility of 0.7 out of 1); the extra year of life begins one year after receiving the intervention. The left-hand column shows the result of a CEA that does not take account of quality of life or time preference. By this analysis, the intervention, which costs $10,000, has a cost-effectiveness of $10,000 per life year gained. The right-hand column shows the result of a CEA that takes account of the suboptimal quality of life produced by the intervention and the year-long delay before the patient receives health benefits. By this analysis, the value of the additional year is discounted by 30% for loss of quality of life (hence it is multiplied by 0.7) and by 3% for the time delay (hence it is multiplied by $1 \div 1.03 = 0.971$),

Without regard to utility or time preference:

$10,000 per life-year (LY)

Incorporating utility and time preference:

$10,000/LY × 0.7 × 0.971
or
$10,000 per 0.679 QALYs
or
$14,712 per QALY

Figure 10.1
Cost-effectiveness of a $10,000 intervention that produces one additional year of health, with a utility of 0.7, occurring one year after receiving the intervention.

resulting in a cost-effectiveness ratio for the intervention of $14,712 per QALY.

As this example shows, CEA is able to accommodate values for quality of life improvement and time discounting into its measurements. In the same way, it could potentially incorporate other values. As we have seen, it currently calculates the number of dollars per quality-adjusted life-year with a discount factor that adjusts for the time period in which the benefits are received:

CEA = $ ÷ (duration of benefit × utility gain × discount rate).

We could add other variables to this equation. For example, suppose we decide that health benefits for women deserve more priority than those for men. We could add a new factor into the equation that increased the value for women's health benefits compared with men's. Similarly, the value of QALYs received could be altered depending on the age of patients receiving the health benefits:

CEA = $ ÷ (duration of benefit × utility gain × discount rate × gender adjuster × age factor × . . .).

This equation is obviously a simplification. It may not always be straightforward simply to add new terms to the cost-effectiveness equation. However, my main point is that many values could potentially be incorporated into CEA once mathematical and other issues are worked out.

Given continuing criticism that CEA does not accurately capture public values for how to set health care priorities, we must look for ways of expanding its value measurement. The challenge is to identify important societal values that are not presently captured to see if CEA can be modified to incorporate them.

Two Values that May Merit Incorporation into CEA

In previous chapters I described two values that could potentially be incorporated into CEA. Let me briefly review them.

Priority to Severely Ill Patients

Because CEA measurement is concerned only with the number of QALYs brought by treatment, it does not address the severity of illness of patients who receive treatment. This contradicts many people's desires to give priority to these patients, even when they gain fewer QALYs than others. Given the rejection of Oregon's CEA list on the grounds that it ignored the rule of rescue, this preference is plausibly a value that deserves to be incorporated into CEA.

Avoiding Discrimination Against People with Limited Treatment Potential Due to Disabilities

QALY measurement has been accused of discriminating against people with disabilities (Hadorn 1992b). Indeed, Oregon's Medicaid rationing plan ran into trouble when its use of quality of life measurement was accused of violating the Americans with Disabilities Act (Sullivan 1992). The emphasis on maximizing QALYs in CEA conflicts with the attitude of some toward saving the lives of people with moderate disabilities (Harris 1987; LaPuma & Lowler 1990; Nord 1993a).

Given the amount of criticism CEA has received for how it handles people with disabilities and the potential that some of its measures may place less value on these lives (Harris 1987), it is worth while to explore whether CEA can be modified so that the value it places on the treatment potential of these people will reflect public sentiment more accurately.

An Obstacle to Incorporating these Two Values into CEA: The QALY Trap

Public preference for giving priority to severely ill patients could easily be incorporated into CEA by rescaling utility measures. If we really

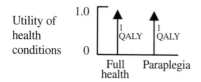

Figure 10.2
Reillustration of the two life-saving treatment programs, assuming the utility of paraplegia is the same as full health.

thought that a change in utility from 0.1 to 0.2 (on a scale of 0 to 1) was twice as important as a change from 0.7 to 0.8, we could rescale utility measures so that the conditions were given a value of 0.1 and 0.3 respectively. In effect, we could stretch out the difference in utility for severe conditions near the bottom of the scale and compress the difference in utility for less severe conditions near the top of the scale.

But this would not allow us to incorporate the second value we discussed. Suppose the public thinks saving the lives of people with paraplegia is equally important as saving the lives of people who can be returned to full health. Then CEA would accommodate this value by rating paraplegia as having the same utility as full health, so that saving the life of both groups would have equal QALYs (figure 10.2). However, this would create two problems. First, within the current conceptual structure of CEA, it would ask us to agree that people with paraplegia have the same quality of life as people without paraplegia. Many would not accept this notion. Second, and more important, it would force us to conclude that curing paraplegia has no medical benefit because it would have no utility. Since the best we can do is to hope to improve the condition so that paraplegics have full health, and since full health and paraplegia have the same utility value according to this revised model, curing paraplegia would not improve utility!

With present methods for measuring cost-effectiveness, we cannot say that saving the life of a paraplegic is equally important as saving the life of a person who can be returned to full health, while simultaneously saying that curing paraplegia is beneficial. This is so because, in the standard approach to QALYs, the utility of a health condition determines not only the benefit of curing it but also the benefit of saving the life of

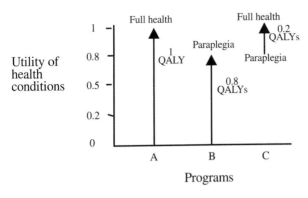

Figure 10.3
The QALY trap: the sum of the treatment value of programs B and C must be
equal to the value of program A.

someone with it. If paraplegia has a utility of 0.8 for the individual,
saving the life of a person with paraplegia for a year (program B in figure
10.3) is judged to bring 0.8 QALYs, and curing the person for a year
(program C) is judged to bring 0.2 QALYs.

The QALY model has us trapped (Nord 1993c). We must decide
whether saving the life of a person with paraplegia is equally important
as saving anyone else's life, or whether instead curing paraplegia brings
some benefit.

A Method to Incorporate Preferences for Severity and
Nondiscrimination into CEA . . . and to Escape the QALY Trap

The value people place on health care programs is determined not only
by the change in QALYs brought by the programs, but also by how
severely ill the patients are who receive the programs and by their
treatment potential. If so, what matters for CEA should not be the change
in individual utility brought by programs but, instead, the *societal value*
people place on the health care programs, which will be determined by
both the expected change in people's health-related utility and by other
considerations.

The QALY trap exists because utility measurement is asked to capture
not only patients' quality of life, but the societal value of treating patients
with various health conditions. When utility measures are supplemented

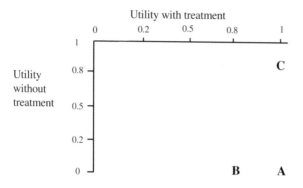

Figure 10.4
Reillustration of treatment programs A, B, and C from figure 10.3

with separate societal value measures, we will no longer be caught in the trap.

The term "societal value" refers to the strength of public preferences for giving priority to various competing health care programs (Nord 1995; Nord et al. 1995). If people think, all else equal, that more severely ill patients should receive priority over less severely ill patients, programs directed toward severely ill patients have greater societal value. An example will illustrate the distinction between how health care programs affect utility and the societal value of those programs.

Figure 10.4 shows programs A, B, and C, which were initially shown in figure 10.3, except now they are represented on a two-dimensional axis, where the vertical axis corresponds to the utility of patients without treatment and the horizontal axis corresponds to the utility they would have with treatment. Program A, which saves people's lives and returns them to full health, is in the lower right hand corner, since these patients would have a utility of zero without treatment and a utility of 1 with treatment (Nord 1992).

Suppose the maximum societal value of any program is given an arbitrary value of 1. Program A will have a societal value of 1 because it brings the greatest possible improvement in utility (ignoring health conditions worse than death for the purpose of this discussion). Now, suppose people think that program B, which saves the lives of people with paraplegia, should receive the same priority for funding as program

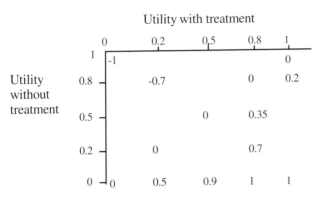

Figure 10.5
Hypothetical societal value matrix illustrating programs A, B, and C and of a series of other health programs.

A. That is, if society could pay to provide ten patients with program A or ten patients with program B, people would be unable to choose which one should receive the funding. In such case, program B would also have a societal value of 1. If people think program C is 1/5 as important as program A, it will have a societal value of 0.2. Figure 10.5 shows a hypothetical example of the societal values of programs A, B, and C and of a series of other programs.

The person trade-off (PTO) method is one possible way to measure societal values. In this method people might be asked how many patients have to be cured of paraplegia (program C) to be equally important as curing ten people of a life-threatening illness and returning them to full health (program A). Suppose someone thought that forty people cured of paraplegia was less beneficial than saving ten people's lives and that curing sixty people of paraplegia was more beneficial, but was unable to decide whether it was better to cure fifty people of paraplegia or save ten people's lives. In this case, a program that cures paraplegia, program C, has 1/5 of the societal value of a program that saves people's lives and returns them to perfect health, program A. There may be other feasible ways of measuring societal values, but utility measurements are *not* acceptable. The key component of societal value measurement, as distinguished from utility measurement, is that it attempts to capture the importance people place on treatment programs relative to other treatment programs when vying for scarce health care resources. Utility measurement would be acceptable only if the value people placed on treatment programs was directly and solely related to the health-related utility brought by the programs.

What is the benefit of separating societal value from utility measurement? As shown in figure 10.3, because of the QALY trap, the total health-related utility brought by programs B and C (in conventional CEA) must add to 1 QALY. However, in the two-dimensional matrix shown in figures 10.4 and 10.5, the societal value of programs B and C does not add to 1 but to 1.2. The values in the matrix are limited so that no single program can have a societal value greater than 1, and so that all programs in which patients receive no improvement in their utility will have a societal value of zero.

Currently, CEA calculates the average change in utility brought by a health care intervention by taking the change in utility of outcomes after the intervention and multiplying this by the probability of each outcome. An intervention that improves utility by 0.1 units in half of a group of patients and by 0.2 units in the other half brings $(0.5 \times 0.1) + (0.5 \times 0.2) = 0.15$ QALYs. The societal value approach is similar, except it replaces the change in utility brought by interventions with the societal value of these changes. This is an important advance because it recognizes that not all similarly sized changes in utility are equally valuable. The value of health care programs is not a simple linear function of how they change utility. It also depends where on the utility scale the changes occur.

By incorporating societal value measures into CEA, we solve the two problems identified earlier. First, we can account for the priorities the general public places on helping severely ill patients. I chose the hypothetical data shown in figure 10.5 to illustrate how a societal value matrix might account for this preference. Health care interventions that improve people's average utility from 0.2 to 0.8, an improvement that only brings 0.6 QALYs per year, are given a societal value of 0.7. In other words, this specific change in utility has a greater value than would be accounted for in traditional CEA.

Second, by incorporating societal value measures into CEA, we can account for public attitudes toward the importance of helping patients who have limited treatment potential because of preexisting disability or chronic illness. Figure 10.5 shows that the value of saving the life of a person with paraplegia is equal to that of saving someone who could be returned to perfect health, despite the reduced utility of paraplegia. It also shows data for life-saving treatments that affect people with more severe disabilities, with utilities of 0.2 and 0.5, respectively. In these two cases, I specify societal values of less than 1 to highlight an important point: societal value measurement does not force us to conclude that saving the life of a person with disability is always equally valuable as saving anyone else. The value of these treatments can be determined only by collecting societal value data. The important point for my purpose is that societal value measurement allows the general public to place greater priority on saving the lives of people with disabilities or chronic illnesses than could be accounted for in traditional CEA measurement, while at the same time allowing significant benefit from curing those disabilities and illnesses.

Some may wonder why the upper left portion of the societal value matrix in figure 10.5 includes negative numbers. Programs in this portion all reduce patients' utility. Why would anyone choose health care interventions that do this? The answer is simple. Most interventions, even when they improve the average utility of a group of patients, decrease utility in some patients. Thus, we have to estimate the societal value of interventions when they worsen utility. In traditional CEA, for example, an intervention that decreases utility by 0.1 in half of patients and increases it by 0.2 in the other half yields an average gain of $(0.5)(0.2)$ + (0.5) (-0.1) = 0.05 QALYs. A similar mathematical weighting would be used in the societal value approach, except utility measures would be replaced by societal value measures.

Some may worry that the societal value approach to QALYs is incoherent because it allows the value of programs B and C to sum to a value greater than 1. Nevertheless, if society places the same value on saving the life of a paraplegic and saving the life of a nonparaplegic, and if society also values the cure of paraplegia, this approach is consistent with societal values. At worst, it is societal values, and not this model, that are inconsistent. However, I do not think societal values in this case would be inconsistent. When people think about the value of saving the life of a person with paraplegia, they are making a separate judgment than when they think about the value of curing paraplegia. Each judgment is made in a different context and at a different time. When they decide about the benefit of curing paraplegia, it is irrelevant what value they think should be placed on saving the life of a person with paraplegia. It is only with a strictly utilitarian set of values, applied with no regard to context, that the suggested procedure can be considered to be inconsistent.

Obstacles to Societal Value Measurement

Societal value measurement is the new kid on the cost-effectiveness block. And cost-effectiveness itself is a relatively new part of town, with many methodological issues about how to measure it still under development. Therefore, we should not be surprised at the many obstacles that could limit its ultimate role in CEA.

In several studies my colleagues and I found a systematic inconsistency in people's PTO responses, which we call *multiplicative intransitivity* (Ubel et al. 1996c). Imagine a person who thinks that curing one person of condition A is equally beneficial as curing ten people of condition B, and that curing one person of condition B is equally beneficial as curing ten of condition C. To be consistent, this person ought to think that curing 1 person of condition A is equally beneficial as curing 100 people of condition C (figure 10.6).

However, when we conducted PTO measurements for three such conditions and multiplied the PTO values of the two "nearer comparisons" (such as A vs B and B vs C), we calculated a different value for the relative importance of the "far comparisons" (such as programs A and C) than people told us when they were directly asked to compare these programs. For example, the same person who said that one person cured of A is equal to ten people being cured of B, and that one person cured of B is the same as ten people cured of C, might say that curing one person of A is equally beneficial as curing fifty people of C.

Well, which is it? Is providing one person with program A equally beneficial as providing fifty people with program C, as the person said? Or does providing 1 person with A bring the same benefit as providing 100 people with C, as we would predict from this person's direct com-

1 person cured of A	=	10 people cured of B
1 person cured of B	=	10 people cured of C
1 person cured of A	=	100 people cured of C

Figure 10.6
Three multiplicatively transitive treatment programs.

parisons of programs A and B and B and C? Whereas measurement error is common in any kind of elicitation task, this error was of concern because it was systematic—the multiplication of nearer values was almost always larger than the direct measure. This type of systematic inconsistency raises fundamental questions about PTO elicitations. Further research is necessary to find out whether these inconsistencies are persistent, or whether they can be corrected through improvement in how PTO questions are asked.

Without a doubt, societal value measurement questions, such as PTO elicitations, are very difficult questions for people to answer. Not many of us have spent a whole lot of time thinking about how many people have to be cured of paraplegia to equal the benefit of saving ten people's lives. Myriad other issues must be resolved before societal value measurement can be incorporated into CEA. But even if societal value measurement in specific, and PTO measurement in particular, are not feasible, the crucial point to remember is that CEA can still be modified to incorporate other values. For example, much the way a discount rate is factored into CEA to capture people's preferences for receiving benefits now rather than later, a severity weight could be factored in to give greater value to health care interventions directed at severely ill patients (Nord et al. 1999).

The Limits of CEA Modification

Although CEA could potentially be modified to account for the two values discussed above, it may never be able to incorporate other values held by the general public. Most important, I do not, at present, see a good way to incorporate concerns for the distribution of health (or health care). As shown in the previous chapter, people care about distributive issues and are willing to give up some health care benefits to distribute the goods more equally, but CEA cannot completely incorporate this value. No matter which factors are added, such as age weights or severity weights, CEA will still show only how to maximize average health. For example, suppose a severity weight was added, resulting in severity-adjusted QALYs. While maximizing severity-adjusted QALYs will have different distributive implications than maximizing traditional QALYs, and while the distribution of health care goods after the adjustment may be more in line with community values, CEA will still show us only how to maximize average severity-adjusted QALYs. If these can be maximized by giving health care services to half of a population instead of an entire population, so be it.

Some may wonder whether distributive concerns could be addressed by factoring in some kind of distribution weight (Keeney & Winkler 1985; Sarin 1985). Any QALYs gained by directing services to a small portion of a population would be discounted compared with those gained by directing services to an entire population. Policy experts have developed mathematical measures of equity so that the relative equity of policy alternatives can be estimated and given a value (Broome 1991; Culyer 1989; Keeney & Winkler 1985; Sarin 1985; Williams 1988). Measuring distributional equity in this way is a promising method of improving certain types of public policy decisions. For example, in deciding about a new environmental regulation, it is not only important to understand how the regulation would affect overall health, but also to understand how those health effects would be distributed. A regulation that causes tiny detriments in many people's health may be preferred to one that causes extreme health problems in a small number of people.

These equity measures, however, do not transfer easily or quickly into health care CEA. When making a major public policy decision about an environmental law or about building a nuclear power plant, it is reasonable to conduct an extensive, one-time economic analysis that looks at, among other things, equity issues. In contrast, CEAs are not intended for a single use but are meant to guide a whole range of medical decisions, from a single hospital's purchasing decisions to federal government decisions about reimbursement for new technologies. Because they are used in so many contexts, it is impossible to model the distributional equity of specific health care interventions.

In one context, a health care system may face budget limits, forcing it to choose between offering the best available treatment to a portion of its patients or a less effective treatment to everyone. Another health care system, with fewer budget constraints, may face no such trade-off between equity and efficiency for these two treatments, but instead may be able to offer the best available treatment to everyone. As this example demonstrates, it makes little sense to calculate distributional equity coefficients for specific interventions. Instead, distributional equity measures are best applied to policy decisions where the distributional effects of available policies on a specific population can be estimated. Since CEA is often used to evaluate specific interventions, such as diagnostic tests and treatment modalities, that will be used in a wide range of settings, such equity concerns are not estimable. Moreover, even if a distributional equity coefficient could be added to CEA, it would vary for each individual or group making use of the cost-effectiveness data, an impossible burden for all but the largest users.

We should not be discouraged that CEA cannot incorporate every potentially important public rationing preference. Even a United States Public Health Service task force, convened to standardize CEA measurement, stated that, at most, CEA was a *guide* to decision making, not the sole determinant of health care decisions (Gold et al. 1996). Our goal should not be to perfect the imperfectable. Instead, it should be to improve what is already a useful decision guide, and one that can be made even more useful if it more closely captures public rationing preferences.

Conclusion

In the future, CEA has tremendous potential to help governments, managed care organizations, insurers, and clinicians rationing at the bedside (!) set health care priorities in a rational and accountable way. However, it has not gained widespread acceptance among decision makers at most of these levels. Part of the reason for this is because CEA does not account for many values that are important to people in how they would choose to set health care priorities, and it is unlikely that it will ever account for every relevant value. Nevertheless, if it is to gain more widespread use in this regard, it should do a better job of capturing relevant public values. Even if used merely as a guide to decision making, we ought to do everything we can to improve how CEA is measured. A promising way to do this is to look more closely at the societal value people place on health care programs and not merely focus on how programs affect people's own individually assessed health-related quality of life.

Certainly, CEA is flawed. It does not capture how people want to ration health care. It ignores fairness and equity to show us how to maximize health, even though most people think maximizing health should not be the sole goal of health care spending. Yet, despite its flaws, CEA deserves an important role in rationing decisions. After all, even if health maximization is not the *sole* goal of health care spending, it is certainly an important one. Moreover, CEA can be improved so that its measures do a better job of reflecting some of the trade-offs between equity and efficiency.

Numbers can be persuasive, and CEA provides numerical estimates that potentially have great psychological effects on health care decision makers. It will be hard for equity considerations to be given equal attention without some attempt to quantify equity. I have tried to show that some equity concerns may be quantifiable in ways that allow them to be incorporated directly into CEA. Alternatively, some may prefer to calculate them separately from CEA so that decision makers can look at both types of numbers.

No matter what we do, we should work hard to provide decision makers with more information about the equity and efficiency of health care interventions so that rationing decisions, whether made at the bedside or in the board room, can better reflect the way people want to balance them.

11
The Future of Cost-Effectiveness Analysis and Health Care Rationing

Cost-effectiveness analysis has had, at best, a troubled youth. To many people, measuring cost-effectiveness is pure folly because, in their minds, health care rationing is unnecessary. If rationing is unnecessary, so is cost-effectiveness. However, to others, even though health care rationing is seen as necessary, CEA is not considered up to the task of telling us how to do it.

But what about the future? Will CEA's troubled youth give way to a successful adulthood? Will people become more aware of the need to ration health care and thus require more of the kind of information CEA provides? Will CEA measurement change so that it can guide our rationing decisions better?

Back to the Future

To see the future of health care rationing, we have only to look at the recent past. In recent years, new drugs for adult-onset diabetes were developed that will potentially control patients' blood sugar without causing weight gain (a significant side effect of previous treatments). But these agents are extremely expensive, and it will be years before we know how much they actually improve people's health. In the past several years, new drugs such as protease inhibitors dramatically improved the health of people infected with HIV, but at such a great financial expense that state-sponsored drug assistance programs, set up to help low-income patients receive therapy ran out of money. Many such programs even instituted rationing guidelines to determine which people would receive which agents. More recently, Viagra revolutionized the care of men with impotence but, again, at an almost staggering financial cost. These new treatments, all released in the past few years, dramatically altered my general internal medicine practice and strengthened my confidence that health care rationing is here to stay. Undoubtedly other advances similarly affected other types of practitioners.

A closer look at recent controversy over payment for Viagra will reveal why health care rationing is only going to grow in upcoming years.

Viagra was introduced in the United States in 1998, first causing a flurry of excitement about the benefits of treating male impotence, and then causing a flurry of press coverage highlighting decisions by insurers about whether to pay for it (Olmos 1998). Public pressure to pay for the drug was great because it was such an improvement over other impotence treatments (Goldstein et al. 1998). But, at $10 a pill, Viagra had the potential to bankrupt insurance companies and managed care organizations. Some third-party payers tried to camouflage this debate by discussing the agent's unproved safety and by debating whether they should be paying to help people have sex. But others were quite willing to admit that the only problem with Viagra was that it cost too much and that they could not afford to offer it to everyone who could benefit from it. Development of this mediagenic compound forced the public to recognize that health care resources are limited.

The attention given to insurers' decisions about whether to pay for Viagra stimulated public debate about which health care services ought to be included in basic benefits packages. Debates such as this, if they continue, will force the public, politicians, and health care providers to decide which services ought to be offered to everyone regardless of their ability to pay, and which should be offered only to those able to pay for them out of pocket. Indeed, the introduction of Viagra for the treatment of impotence, and protease inhibitors for the treatment of HIV-related illness, give us a window into the future of health care rationing. Although the view through this window is cloudy, enough of the future is clear to predict a few things about bedside rationing, CEA, and the general need to ration health care.

New Medical Advances Will Increase the Pressure on Third-Party Payers to Ration Health Care Implicitly

When new medical advances arrive, third-party payers often feel great pressure to pay for them. Consequently, these advances fuel health care inflation (Callahan, 1998). Third-party payers could reduce such inflationary effects by limiting the use of other health care services. Every dollar spent on Viagra, for example, could be taken away from some other medical expenditure. But it is rare for third-party payers to set explicit limits on services that were previously available to all. I know of none that explicitly came out and stated how they would save money to make up for the additional expense of Viagra. Not one said, for example, that they would pay for Viagra, but would stop paying for lung transplants, PSA tests, physical therapy, or titanium hip prostheses.

It is true that when protease inhibitors became available, AIDS drug assistance programs had to make explicit decisions about whether to offer them and, if so, which other drugs to remove from their formularies to pay for them. But these programs are not typical third-party payers, at least in the United States, and they face specific budgetary constraints. When they exhaust their budget on expensive drugs, they simply run out of money and must stop providing treatment until the next fiscal year arrives. In contrast, most third-party payers in this country do not have specific budget limits. Thus they have typically provided protease inhibitors to patients without making any explicit public decisions about how they will pay for the agents. How do third-party payers afford expensive new medical advances?

Occasionally, a medical advance arrives that improves health and saves money, but most only improve people's health at a financial cost. This leaves third-party payers with two basic options:

1. Refuse to pay for the new intervention.
2. Pay for the intervention, at least for some patients.

Option 1 is rarely taken. Most new advances have an identifiable interest group lobbying to make the service available to patients in need. Sometimes patients themselves organize lobbying groups. Perhaps more often, physicians lobby third-party payers to reimburse for the advances.

In the VA health care system, a group of neurologists urged the system to pay for new drugs to treat Parkinson's disease. These clinicians had the best interests of patients in mind and believed that the agents were an important advance in their treatment.

This leaves option 2—pay for the intervention. When third-party payers choose this, they have several ways to cover the additional expense:

2a. By accepting reduced profits or a reduction in their financial bottom line.

2b. By increasing health insurance premiums.

2c. By saving money on other interventions to maintain budget neutrality.

Option 2a is, at best, a temporary fix. Third-party payers can lose money only for so long. As new advances arrive, they must choose either option 2b or option 2c.

But haven't I already ruled out option 2c? Haven't I already said that third-party payers are unwilling explicitly to limit previously available services to pay for new ones?

True, I did say that third-party payers are unlikely *explicitly* to limit services, but that does not mean I have ruled out the option, because third-party payers can still limit services by rationing them *implicitly*. They do not have to make public announcements about how they will pay for new agents such as Viagra. Instead, they simply have to increase pressure on clinicians, home health care agencies, hospitals, and other health care providers to do more with less.

When third-party payers adopt new medical advances as standard of care, they do not generally do so at the explicit public expense of other available interventions. Instead, the advances will increase health care costs, will increase implicit health care rationing, or, perhaps most often, will increase health care costs at the same time that they increase pressure to ration health care implicitly.

Reliance on Implicit Health Care Rationing Will Increase Pressure on Clinicians to Ration at the Bedside

The unwillingness of third-party payers in the United States to say explicitly how they will contain health care costs means that the only way to decrease the inflationary effects of expensive medical advances is through implicit rationing. This will increase pressure on clinicians to ration at the bedside. If third-party payers increase their use of utilization review, this will increase bedside rationing because clinicians will eventually have to decide whether to accept the recommendations of the reviewers. If third-party payers increase their use of capitation, as I have already stated, this will succeed only through bedside rationing.

Even when third-party payers are willing explicitly to ration health care, they will still rely, at least in part, on bedside rationing. Outside the United States, many governments rely on relatively fixed budgets to control health care spending. Often, the spending limits are well known, which makes clinicians more likely to accept bedside rationing. For example, 87% of physicians surveyed in the United Kingdom agreed that "rationing of prescribed drugs should take the form of individual clinical decisions as part of the general practitioner-patient relationship, rather than depending on whether the practice has over or under spent its prescribing budget" (Baines, Tolley, & Whynes 1998). In short, not only is rationing here to stay, bedside rationing is here to stay, too.

How Should Clinicians Decide Which Services to Ration at the Bedside?

I emphasized the need for clinicians rationing at the bedside to identify marginally beneficial services that produce small benefits at large financial costs. In addition, I suggested that CEA is a promising way to identify these services. But I also spent several chapters discussing moral and methodologic problems with CEA.

Given these limitations, what should clinicians do? How should they go about identifying marginally beneficial services they can appropriately withhold from their patients?

I have no perfect answers to these questions. Nevertheless, several points are worth keeping in mind as clinicians struggle with these decisions.

First, despite its imperfections, CEA is a good place to start when trying to identify marginally beneficial services to ration. It gives clinicians a reference point to compare and judge interventions. With so many beneficial interventions available, CEAs give us an idea about how much money we must spend to achieve a certain amount of benefit. Thus, clinicians should familiarize themselves with how to interpret them, and medical schools, nursing schools, and clinical training programs should add such courses to their curricula. It is as important for clinicians to know something about the basic science of CEA measurement as it is to know about the basic science of the Krebs cycle, and probably more important than it is to know the Latin terms they are forced to memorize in anatomy class.

Second, clinicians have to be aware of CEA's limitations, especially its moral limitations. As I discussed previously, CEA undervalues the benefits of life-saving treatments and of interventions directed at improving the health of people with severe illness or disability. Thus, if a life-saving therapy is equally cost effective as a nonlife-saving therapy, the former is probably more important to the public. If the cost-effectiveness of intensive care treatment for a life-threatening disease is equal to that of a life-saving screening test, the former is probably more important. When a little girl falls in a well, no one asks how much money it will take to get her out. We simply do what we can to save her. The public places special importance on directing resources to identifiably and desperately ill patients.

Indeed, bedside rationing is inappropriate when deciding whether to offer life-saving treatments to specific patients. This is an important point, so let me elaborate. In recent years, significant debate has centered on whether doctors can ever morally justify refusing a life-saving treatment to a patient on the grounds that it is futile. Experts disagree about what chance of success qualifies as "futile" (Lantos et al. 1989; Schneiderman, Jecker, & Jonsen 1990; Truog, Brett, & Frader 1992). They agree that interventions with *no* chance of success are futile, but these are extremely rare. Whereas intensive care unit (ICU) care for someone recently decapitated is obviously futile, most of the time it is impossible to say that it has zero percent chance of success. No series of similar cases will prove that the next case will turn out the same way, so even if the last 100 patients admitted to the ICU with a similar illness died (Schneiderman et al. 1990), the next one may survive.

However, one concept has been virtually absent from debates about futility—economics (Jecker & Schneiderman 1992). This absence is informative. Although it is difficult to define what percentage chance of success is futile, most interventions that approach zero percent are extremely cost ineffective. If ICU treatment has less than 1% chance of benefiting a patient, at a cost of tens of thousands of dollars per patient treated, the math is not too difficult. The cost per year of life saved will be extremely high. Nevertheless, few people have wanted to frame futility debates in economic terms. This is in large part because most people do not think decisions about whether to attempt life-saving therapy for identifiably ill patients should be based on cost. In contrast, decisions about whether to adopt new but expensive advances in Pap smear technology are based solely on cost-effectiveness.

In short, when deciding whether to offer specific patients potentially life-saving surgery, ICU care, or other such treatments, society has decided, rightly or wrongly, that money should not influence decisions. Thus, in these settings, it would be inappropriate to ration at the bedside. Instead, decisions should be based on the balance of burdens and benefits to the patients, based on patients' values whenever possible. If rationing is to occur when deciding whether to offer expensive, potentially life-saving treatment to an identifiably ill patient, it should not be done at the bedside; it should not be based on the discretion of an individual clinician. Instead, this decision should be made at a higher level by a health care system or government. It should be based on some kind of community consensus that this type of patient should not receive this expensive treatment.

I do not mean to suggest that bedside rationing should be absent from ICUs. It can occur many times in these settings, such as in daily decisions about whether to order certain blood tests or radiographs. But it is inappropriate when deciding whether to admit a specific patient to the ICU, not in deciding whether a low-yield diagnostic test is worth while to do once the patient has been admitted.

I once took over the care of a man whose previous primary care physician had tried to withhold blood products from him on the basis that this gentleman's quality of life was not good enough to justify his transfusion needs. The man was seriously ill with severe congestive heart failure and a chronic bleeding disorder in his colon. He was an ornery man, and his family was even worse; many of his family members had been in and out of penal institutions, and rumor had it that they were trying to keep him alive only so they could collect his disability checks.

Although this patient was incredibly challenging to care for, it was totally inappropriate for this clinician to ration blood products from him. I do not know how cost-effective it was to transfuse this patient. But I do know that his wife shared a bed with him, even though he was frequently incontinent of urine and stool. No disability check would compel most of us to do that. And I also know that this man and his wife loved each other very much, and that it was important for them to be with each other as long as possible. So even though this man's quality of life looked dismal to many clinicians taking care of him, he still enjoyed his life very much. When trying to conserve medical resources, clinicians must be very cautious making judgments about whether a specific patient's quality of life is good enough to deserve resources.

Contrast the clinician in this case with one who decides not to prescribe cholesterol-lowering drugs for patients at low risk of developing heart disease. Evidence is accumulating that most of us could decrease our risk of heart attack by taking one of these agents. But people at low risk of developing heart disease—those without a family history of heart disease, who are not obese, and do not have high blood pressure or diabetes— receive these benefits infrequently (Pearson 1998). If a person has only a 1% lifetime chance of heart disease, therapy cannot reduce the heart attack risk by a very large amount. For these low-risk people, the cost-effectiveness of cholesterol reduction is dismal. Clinicians who decide not to push for cholesterol reduction in these people will save the health care system significant money, while having only a small effect on the health of the population. These clinicians are not making life-and-death decisions based on a patient's perceived quality of life. They are making population-based decisions (with some attention to patients' specific circumstances) about whether scarce health care dollars are best spent on preventing heart attacks in people unlikely to have them.

Another consideration is in order when rationing at the bedside: clinicians have to pay attention to the organizational context of their decisions. Rationing within the VA system is different than rationing at a for-profit health care company. This affects the justifiability and appropriateness of decisions. (Indeed, clinicians have to be much more aggressive about debating institutional rationing policies and financial policies. If health care companies want to maximize profits aggressively, clinicians must step in to remind the institution of other priorities!)

Whereas I have tried to provide some guidance about how to ration at the bedside, most issues have not been sorted out satisfactorily. For example, the role of informed consent in bedside rationing is not well understood. Research might illuminate how well clinicians can discuss these issues with patients and whether such discussions improve or harm clinician-patient relationships. But in the meantime, clinicians must decide for themselves how and when to discuss cost-containment efforts with patients. We have been debating whether rationing is necessary for so long that we have not spent much time discussing how to do it. Ultimately, clinicians have to decide for themselves what their threshold is for offering small benefits to patients, and when they should discuss patients' out-of-pocket costs. But, with time, this personal judgment should be informed by rational public debate, and even data, about bedside rationing.

The Future of Health Care Rationing and Cost-Effectiveness Analysis

I predicted that medical advances will increase health care inflation and thereby increase implicit health care rationing, especially bedside rationing. But some rationing decisions will clearly be made at higher administrative levels, above that of the individual clinician encountering a specific patient. How will the health care system ration?

I am not an expert on organizational or management theory, and do not know enough about politics, either, to pretend to say how health care systems will ration. Instead, I want to put in a final word for how they *ought* to ration. Researchers have to find ways to improve their understanding of how the general public wants to ration health care, with specific attention to which preferences deserve to be incorporated into policy decisions, to help guide well-intended third-party payers when making these decisions.

Of course, public preferences alone should not determine how we ration health care. Some members of the general public may not want to give health care services to homosexuals with AIDS or to alcoholics with liver disease. As philosopher John Rawls (1971) wrote:

> The intense convictions of the majority, if they are indeed mere preferences without any foundation in the principles of justice antecedently established, have no weight to begin with. The satisfaction of these feelings has no value that can be put in the scales against the claims of equal liberty.

Public preferences can be unjust, and therefore the way we incorporate them into health care rationing should be constrained by principles of justice. We do not want a system ruled by a tyranny of the majority. This is potentially a place where government regulation can play an important role in setting boundaries. In the United States, laws such as the Americans with Disabilities Act potentially prevent health care institutions from devising policies that discriminate against disabled people.

But the government and other third-party payers require better research from ethicists and experts in measuring community values. To ration justly, ethicists, economists, psychologists, sociologists, clinicians, and others must get together to determine which decisions would be improved by more public input. A couple of the examples in this book are good candidates. Reasonable people (even reasonable philosophers) can disagree about how much priority we should give to severely ill patients. Thus, we should find out how much priority the public wants to give to such patients and base policy decisions in part on these preferences. In contrast, most ethicists would not endorse a rationing system based on whether patients regularly attend church. We should not look to the general public in such cases to see whether they want to base decisions on such social worth criteria.

Where might CEA fit into the picture? I predict that CEA, or something much like it, is here for the long haul. Too many rationing decisions have to be made to ignore the power of this economic information. So far, the role of CEA has been limited, but, then, measuring cost effectiveness in health care is a relatively recent phenomenon. Twenty years ago, no one did it, so it is not surprising that CEA has yet to wield significant influence over rationing decisions.

My hope is that cost-effectiveness information will play an increasing role in rationing decisions. My dream is that CEA measurement will be modified to incorporate public rationing preferences. My realistic prediction is that administrators, clinicians, and policy experts will become significantly better at interpreting CEAs and increasingly comfortable at basing their decisions in part on cost-effectiveness.

But, whatever happens to CEA measurement, or to the use of CEA in decisions regarding health care rationing, fundamental moral dilemmas will always remain. We will never have an acceptable answer to the question: how much money should we spend to save someone's life? And we will probably never resolve our inconsistencies about the values we place on saving identifiably ill patients versus saving statistical lives through preventive care.

But moral dilemmas do not lose their relevance simply because they are irresolvable. Instead, their irresolvability indicates their continued relevance. We must never stop debating the price of life. And we must never stop arguing about how much money to spend on health care.

Life is priceless. But health care is expensive, and one way or another, society must decide how much money to spend on it. With luck, these decisions will be informed by economic data about the cost-effectiveness of the remarkable interventions available to those of us in developed countries, and by moral arguments about how we can improve people's health while ensuring that they have fair access to good health care.

References

Aaron, H.J. & W.B. Schwartz. (1990). Rationing health care: The choice before us. *Science* 247, 418–422.

Alderman, M.H. (1992). Which antihypertensive drugs first—And why! *Journal of the American Medical Association* 267, 2786–2787.

Anders, G. (1996). *Health Against Wealth: HMOs and the Breakdown of Medical Trust.* Boston: Houghton Mifflin.

Angell, M. (1985). Cost containment and the physician. *Journal of the American Medical Association* 254, 1203–1207.

Angell, M. (1993). The doctor as double agent. *Kennedy Institute of Ethics Journal* 3, 279–286.

Asch, D.A. & P.A. Ubel. (1997). Rationing by any other name. *New England Journal of Medicine* 336, 1668–1671.

Ayres, I., L.G. Dooley, & R.S. Gaston. (1993). Unequal racial access to kidney transplantation. *Vanderbilt Law Review* 46, 805–863.

Baines, D.L., K.H. Tolley, & D.K. Whynes. (1998). The ethics of resource allocation: The views of general practitioners in Lincolnshire, U.K. *Social Science and Medicine* 47, 1555–1564.

Baker, R. & M.A. Strosberg. (1992). Triage and equality: An historical reassessment of utilitarian analyses of triage. *Kennedy Institute of Ethics Journal* 2, 103–123.

Barber, R.L. (1987). Public policy and the allocation of scarce medical resources. *Journal of Philosophy* 84, 655–665.

Baron, J. (1995). Blind justice: Fairness to groups and the do-no-harm principle. *Journal of Behavioral Decision Making* 8, 71–83.

Baron, J. (1996). Heuristics and biases in equity judgments: A utilitarian approach. In B.A. Mellers & J. Baron (Eds.), *Psychological Perspectives on Justice: Theory and Applications* (pp. 109–137). Cambridge: Cambridge University Press.

Baron, J. & P.A. Ubel. (In press). Inconsistencies in person-tradeoff and difference judgments of health-state utility. *Journal of Experimental Psychology—Applied.*

Barret, B.J., P.S. Parfrey, H.M. Vavasour, et al. (1992). Comparison of nonionic, low-osmolality radiocontrast agents with ionic, high-osmolality agents during cardiac catheterization. *New England Journal of Medicine* 326, 431–436.

Barry, M.J., A.G. Mulley, F.J. Fowler, & J.W. Wennberg. (1988). Watchful waiting vs immediate transurethral resection for symptomatic prostatism: The importance of patients' preferences. *Journal of the American Medical Association* 259, 3010–3017.

Berwick, D.M. & K.L. Coltin. (1986). Feedback reduces test use in a health maintenance organization. *Journal of the American Medical Association* 255, 1450–1454.

Bowling, A. (1996). Health care rationing: The public's debate. *British Medical Journal* 312, 670–674.

Brett, A.S. & L.B. McCullough. (1986). When patients request specific interventions: Defining the limits of the physician's obligation. *New England Journal of Medicine* 315, 1347–1351.

Brook, R.H. (1989). Practice guidelines and practicing medicine: Are they compatible? *Journal of the American Medical Association* 262, 3027–3030.

Brook, R.H. & K.N. Lohr. (1986). Will we need to ration effective health care? *Issues in Science and Technology* Fall, 68–77.

Brook, R.H., J.E. Ware, W.H. Rogers, et al. (1983). Does free care improve adults' health? Results from a randomized controlled trial. *New England Journal of Medicine* 309, 1426–1434.

Broome, J. (1991). *Weighing Goods*. Oxford: Blackwell.

Bryant, J.H. (1973). Human criteria in health care. *Ecumenical Review* 25, 80–86, 91–98.

Bryce, C.L. & K.E. Cline. (1998). The supply and use of selected medical technologies. *Health Affairs* 17, 213–224.

Buchanan, J. & S. Cretin. (1986). Fee-for-service health care expenditures: Evidence of selction effects among subscribers who choose HMOs. *Medical Care* 24, 39–51.

Calabresi, G. & P. Bobbit. (1978). *Tragic Choices: The Conflicts Society Confronts in the Allocation of Tragically Scarce Resources*. New York: W.W. Norton.

Callahan, D. (1987). *Setting Limits: Medical Goals in an Aging Society*. New York: Simon & Schuster.

Callahan, D. (1990). *What Kind of Life: The Limits of Medical Progress*. New York: Simon & Schuster.

Callahan, D. (1998). *False Hopes: Why America's Quest for Perfect Health Is a Recipe for Failure*. New York: Simon & Schuster.

Cassel, C. (1985). Doctors and allocation decisions: A new role in the new Medicare. *Journal of Health Politics, Policy, and Law* 10, 549–564.

Churchill, L.R. (1987). *Rationing Health Care in America: Perceptions and Principles of Justice*. Notre Dame, IN: Notre Dame University Press.

Cohen, J. (1996). Preferences, needs and QALYs. *Journal of Medical Ethics* 22, 267–272.

Collins, M.M. & M.J. Barry. (1996). Controversies in prostate cancer screening. Analogies to the early lung cancer screening debate. *Journal of the American Medical Association* 276, 1976–1979.

Culyer, A.J. (1989). The normative economics of health care finance and provision. *Oxford Review of Economic Policy 5.*

Daniels, N. (1985). *Just Health Care.* Cambridge: Cambridge University Press.

Daniels, N. (1987). The ideal advocate and limited resources. *Theoretical Medicine* 8, 69–80.

Daniels, N. (1991). Is the Oregon rationing plan fair? *Journal of the American Medical Association* 265, 2232–2235.

Daniels, N. (1992). Justice and health care rationing: Lessons from Oregon. In M.A. Strosberg, J.M. Wiener, R. Baker, & I.A. Fein (Eds.), *Rationing America's Medical Care: The Oregon Plan and Beyond.* Washington, DC: Brookings Institution.

Deyo, R.A., B.M. Psaty, G. Simon, et al. (1997). The messenger under attack—Intimidation of researchers by special-interest groups. *New England Journal of Medicine* 336, 1176–1180.

Eddy, D.M. (1990). Screening for cervical cancer. *Annals of Internal Medicine* 113, 214–226.

Eddy, D.M. (1991a). *Common Screening Tests.* Philadelphia: American College of Physicians.

Eddy, D.M. (1991b). Oregon's methods: Did cost-effectiveness fail? *Journal of the American Medical Association* 266, 2135–2141.

Eddy, D.M. (1992a). Applying cost-effectiveness analysis: The inside story. *Journal of the American Medical Association* 268, 2575–2582.

Eddy, D.M. (1992b). Cost-effectiveness analysis: A conversation with my father. *Journal of the American Medical Association* 267, 1669–1675.

Eddy, D.M. (1994). Health system reform: Will controlling costs require rationing services? *Journal of the American Medical Association* 272, 324–328.

Eddy, D.M., F.W. Nugent, J.F. Eddy, et al. (1987). Screening for colorectal cancer in a high-risk population: Results of a mathematical model.

Elster, J. (1992). *Local Justice: How Institutions Allocate Scarce Goods and Necessary Burdens.* New York: Russell Sage Foundation.

Emanuel, E.J. (1991). *The Ends of Human Life: Medical Ethics in a Liberal Polity.* Cambridge: Harvard University Press.

Evans, R.W. (1983). Health care technology and the inevitability of resource allocation and rationing decisions. *Journal of the American Medical Association* 249, 2208–2219.

Fins, J.J. (1998). Drug benefits in managed care: Seeking ethical guidance from the formulary? *Journal of the American Geriatric Society* 46, 346–350.

Fischhoff, B. (1991). Value elicitation: Is there anything in there? *American Psychologist* 46, 835–847.

Fletcher, S.W. (1997). Whither scientific deliberation in health policy recommendations? Alice in the Wonderland of breast-cancer screening. *New England Journal of Medicine* 336, 1180–1183.

Fowler, F.J., D.M. Berwick, A. Roman, & M.P. Massagli. (1994). Measuring public priorities for insurable health care. *Medical Care* 625–639.

Fox, D.M. & H.M. Leichter. (1991). Rationing care in Oregon: The new accountability. *Health Affairs* 10, 7–27.

Froberg, D.G. & R.L. Kane. (1989). Methodology for measuring health-state preferences. II. Scaling methods. *Journal of Clinical Epidemiology* 42, 459–471.

Fryback, D.G. & W.F. Lawrence. (1997). Dollars may not buy as many QALYs as we think: A problem with defining quality-of-life adjustments. *Medical Decision Making* 17, 276–284.

Fuchs, V. (1984). The "rationing" of medical care. *New England Journal of Medicine* 311, 1572–1573.

Fuchs, V.R. (1996). What every philosopher should know about health economics. *Health Economics* 140, 186–195.

Fuchs, V.R. (1998). Ethics and economics: Antagonists or allies in making health policy? *Western Journal of Medicine* 168, 213–216.

Furrow, B.R. (1988). The ethics of cost-containment: Bureaucratic medicine and the doctor as patient-advocate. *Journal of Law, Ethics, and Public Policy* 3, 187–225.

Gal. I. & J. Baron. (1996). Understanding repeated choices. *Thinking and Reasoning* 2, 81–98.

Garland, M.J. (1992). Rationing in public: Oregon's priority-setting methodology. In M.A. Strosberg, J.M. Wiener, R. Baker, & I.A. Fein (Eds.), *Rationing America's Medical Care: The Oregon Plan and Beyond.* Washington, DC: Brookings Institution.

Gaston, R., I. Ayres, L.G. Dooley, & A.G. Diethelm. (1993). Racial equity in renal transplantation: The disparate impact of HLA-based allocation. *Journal of the American Medical Association* 270, 1352–1356.

Gold, M.R., J. Siegel, L.B. Russell, & M. Weinstein. (1996). *Cost-Effectiveness in Health and Medicine.* New York: Oxford University Press.

Goldstein, I., T. Lue, H. Padma-Nathan, et al. (1998). Oral sildenafil in the treatment of erectile dysfunction. *New England Journal of Medicine* 338, 1397–1404.

Goold, S.D. (1998). Money and trust: Physician incentives and the doctor-patient relationship. *Journal of Health, Politics, Policy, and Law* 23, 687–695.

Gramlich, E.M. (1990). *A Guide to Benefit-Cost Analysis.* Englewood Cliffs, NJ: Prentice-Hall.

Griffin, A. & D.C. Thomasma. (1983). Pediatric critical care. *Archives of Internal Medicine* 143, 325.

Grubbs, M.C., H.J. Schultz, N.K. Henry, et al. (1992). Ciprofloxacin versus trimethoprim-sulfamethoxazole: Treatment of community-acquired urinary tract infections in a prospective, controlled, double-blind comparison. *Mayo Clinic Proceedings* 67, 1163–1168.

GUSTO. (1993). An international randomized trial comparing four thrombolytic strategies for acute myocardial infarction. *New England Journal of Medicine* 329, 673–682.

Hadorn, D.C. (1991). Setting health care priorities in Oregon: Cost-effectiveness meets the rule of rescue. *Journal of the American Medical Association* 265, 2218–2225.

Hadorn, D.C. (1992a). *Basic Benefits and Clinical Guidelines*. Boulder, CO: Westview Press.

Hadorn, D.C. (1992b). The problem of discrimination in health care priority setting. *Journal of the American Medical Association* 268, 1454–1459.

Hadorn, D.C. & R.H. Brook. (1991). The health care resource allocation debate: Defining our terms. *Journal of the American Medical Association* 266, 3328–3331.

Hall, M.A. (1994). The problems with rule-based rationing. *Journal of Medicine and Philosophy* 19, 315–332.

Hall, M.A. (1997). Making Medical Spending Decisions: The Law, Ethics, and Economics of Rationing Mechanisms. New York: Oxford University Press.

Hamilton, E. & H. Cairns. (1961). *Plato: The Collected Dialogues, Including the Letters*. Princeton, NJ: Princeton University Press.

Harris, J. (1987). QALYfying the value of life. *Journal of Medical Ethics* 13, 117–123.

Havighurst, C.C. (1992). Prospective self denial: Can consumers contract today to accept health care rationing tomorrow? *University of Pennsylvania Law Review* 140, 1755–1808.

Hiatt, H.H. (1975). Protecting the medical commons: Who is responsible? *New England Journal of Medicine* 293, 235–241.

Hibbard, J.H., J.J. Jewett, S. Engelmann, & M. Tusler. (1998). Can Medicare beneficiaries make informed choices? *Health Affairs* 17, 181–193.

Hillman, A.L. (1987). Financial incentives for physicians in HMOs: Is there a conflict of interest. *New England Journal of Medicine* 317, 1743–1748.

Hillman, A.L. (1990). Health maintenance organizations, financial incentives, and physicians' judgments. *Annals of Internal Medicine* 112, 891–893.

Hillman, A.L., M.V. Pauly, K. Kerman, & C. Rohr. (1991). HMO managers' views on financial incentives and quality. *Health Affairs* 10, 207–219.

Hillman, A.L., M.V. Pauly, & J.J. Kerstein. (1989). How do financial incentives affect physicians' clinical decisions and the financial performance of health maintenance organizations? *New England Journal of Medicine* 321, 86–92.

Hochla, P.K.O. & V.B. Tuason. (1992). Pharmacy and therapeutics committee: Cost-containment considerations. *Archives of Internal Medicine* 152, 1773–1775.

Hornberger, J.C., D.A. Redelmeier, & J. Petersen. (1992). Variability among methods to assess patients' well-being and consequent effect on a cost-effectiveness analysis. *Journal of Clinical Epidemiology* 45, 505–512.

Jackson-Beeck, M. & J.H. Kleinman. (1983). Evidence for self-selection among health maintenance organization enrollees. *Journal of the American Medical Association* 250, 2826–2829.

Jacobson, B. & A. Bowling. (1995). Involving the public: Practical and ethical issues. *British Medical Bulletin* 51, 869–875.

Jecker, N.S. & L.J. Schneiderman. (1992). Futility and rationing. *American Journal of Medicine* 92, 189–196.

Jenni, K.E. & G. Loewenstein. (1997). Explaining the "identifiable victim" effect. *Journal of Risk and Uncertainty* 14, 235–257.

Jonsen, A. (1986). Bentham in a box: Technology assessment and health care allocation. *Law, Medicine and Health Care* 14, 172–174.

Kahneman, D. & J. Snell. (1990). Predicting utility. In R.M. Hogarth (Ed.), *Insights in Decision Making: A Tribute to Hillel J. Einhorn* (pp. 295–310). Chicago and London: University of Chicago Press.

Kahneman, D. & C. Varey. (1991). Notes on the psychology of utility. In J. Elster & J.E. Roemer (Eds.), *Interpersonal Comparisons of Well-Being* (pp. 127–163). Cambridge: Cambridge University Press.

Kaplan, R.M. (1992). A quality-of-life approach to health resource allocation. In M.A. Strosberg, J.M. Wiener, R. Baker, & I.A. Fein (Eds.), *Rationing America's Medical Care: The Oregon Plan and Beyond* (pp. 60–77). Washington, DC: Brookings Institution.

Kassirer, J.P. (1997). Our endangered integrity: It can only get worse. *New England Journal of Medicine* 336, 1666–1667.

Keeler, E.B., J.L. Buchanan, & J.E. Rolph. (1988). *The Demand for Episodes of Treatment in the Health Insurance Experiment*. Santa Monica, CA: Rand Corporation.

Keeney, R.L. & R.L. Winkler. (1985). Evaluating decision strategies for equity of public risks. *Operations Research* 33, 955–970.

Kitzhaber, J.A. (1993). Rationing in action: Prioritising health services in an era of limits: The Oregon experience. *British Medical Journal* 307, 373–377.

Klein, R. (1998). Why Britain is reorganizing its national health service—Yet again. *Health Affairs* 17, 111–125.

Klevit, H.D., A.C. Bates, T. Castanares, et al. (1991). Prioritization of health care services: A progress report by the Oregon Health Services Commission. *Archives of Internal Medicine* 151, 912–916.

Kliger, C.H. (1995). Use of ethical criteria in medical decision making: Corneal transplantation. *Archives of Ophthalmology* 113, 988–993.

Krahn, M. & A. Gafni. (1993). Discounting in the economic evaluation of health care interventions. *Medical Care* 31, 403–418.

Lantos, J.D., P.A. Singer, R.M. Walker, et al. (1989). The illusion of futility in clinical practice. *American Journal of Medicine* 87, 81–84.

LaPuma, J. & E.F. Lawlor. (1990). Quality-adjusted life-years: Ethical implications for physicians and policymakers. *Journal of the American Medical Association* 263, 2917–2921.

Lee, P.R. & A.R. Jonsen. (1974). The right to health care. *American Review of Respiratory Disease* 109, 591–592.

Levinsky, N.G. (1984). The doctor's master. *New England Journal of Medicine* 311, 1573–1575.

Levinsky, N.G. (1998). Truth or consequences. *New England Journal of Medicine* 338, 913–915.

Lipsitch, M. (1995). Fears growing over bacteria resistant to antibiotics. *New York Times* (12 September, p. C1).

Lohr, K.N., R.H. Brook, C.J. Kamberg, et al. (1986). Use of medical care in the Rand health insurance experiment: Diagnosis- and service-specific analyses in a randomized controlled trial. *Medical Care* 24, S1–S87.

Loomes, G. & L. McKenzie. (1989). The use of QALYs in health care decision making. *Social Science and Medicine* 28, 299–308.

Macklin, R. (1993). *Enemies of Patients.* New York: Oxford University Press.

Mandel, J.S., J.H. Bond, M. Bradley, et al. (1993). Reducing mortality from colorectal cancer by screening for fecal occult blood. *New England Journal of Medicine* 328, 1365–1371.

Marsh, F.H. & M. Yarborough. (1990). *Medicine and Money: A Study of the Role of Beneficence in Health Care Cost Containment.* Westport, CT: Greenwold Press.

Maynard, A. & K. Bloor. (1995). Help or hindrance? The role of economics in rationing health care. *British Medical Bulletin* 51, 854–868.

McDonald, C.J., J.M. Overhage, W.M. Tierney, et al. (1996). The promise of computerized feedback systems for diabetes care. *Annals of Internal Medicine* 124, 170–174.

McNeil, B.J., S.G. Pauker, H.C. Sox, & A. Tversky. (1982). On the elicitation of preferences for alternative therapies. *New England Journal of Medicine* 306, 1259–1262.

McPherson, K., J.E. Wennberg, O.B. Hovind, & P. Clifford. (1982). Small-area variations in the use of common surgical procedures: An international comparison of New England, England, and Norway. *New England Journal of Medicine* 307, 1310–1314.

Mechanic, D. (1979). *Future Issues in Health Care, Social Policy and the Rationing of Medical Services.* New York: Free Press.

Mechanic, D. (1992). Professional judgment and the rationing of medical care. *University of Pennsylvania Law Review* 140, 1713–1754.

Menzel, P.T. (1990). *Strong Medicine: The Ethical Rationing of Health Care.* New York: Oxford University Press.

Miles, S. & R. Bendiksen. (1994). Minnesota public opinion on health care resource allocation. *Minnesota Medicine* 77, 19–23.

Mill, J.S. (1973). Utilitarianism. In *The Utilitarians.* Anchor Press/Doubleday. Garden City, NY.

Miller, D. (1976). *Social Justice.* Oxford: Clarendon Press.

Morreim, E.H. (1985). The MD and the DRG. *Hastings Center Report* 15, 30–38.

Moser, M. (1993). Current hypertension management: Separating fact from fiction. *Cleveland Clinic Journal of Medicine* 60, 27–37.

Naylor, C.D. (1991). A different view of queues in Ontario. *Health Affairs* Fall, 110–127.

Neuhauser, D. & A.M. Lewicki. (1976). National health insurance and the sixth stool guaiac. *Policy Analysis* 2, 175–96.

Nord, E. (1991). The validity of a visual analogue scale in determining social utility weights for health states. *International Journal of Health Planning and Management* 6, 234–242.

Nord, E. (1992). An alternative to QALYs: The saved young life equivalent (SAVE). *British Medical Journal* 305, 875–877.

Nord, E. (1993a). The relevance of health state after treatment in prioritising between different patients. *Journal of Medical Ethics* 19, 37–42.

Nord, E. (1993b). The trade-off between severity of illness and treatment effect in cost-value analysis of health care. *Health Policy* 24, 227–238.

Nord, E. (1993c). Unjustified use of the quality of well-being scale in priority setting in Oregon. *Health Policy* 24, 45–53.

Nord, E. (1995). The person trade-off approach to valuing health care programs. *Medical Decision Making* 15, 201–208.

Nord, E., J. Richardson, H. Kuhse, & P. Singer. (1995). Who cares about cost? Does economic analysis impose or reflect social values? *Health Policy* 34, 79–94.

Nord, E., J. Richardson, & K. Macarounas-Kirchmann. (1993). Social evaluation of health care versus personal evaluation of health states: Evidence on the validity of four health-state scaling instruments using Norwegian and Australian surveys. *International Journal of Technology Assessment* 9, 463–478.

Nord, E., J.L. Pinto, J. Richardson, et al. (1999). Incorporating societal concerns for fairness in numerical valuations of health programs. *Health Economics* 8, 25–39.

Olmos, D.R. (1998). Viagra shows the potency of insurers; this drug and other medical breakthroughs raise questions about how companies decide what to cover and how that affects people's lives. *Los Angeles Time* (7 June, (A1.

Olsen, J.A. (1993). On what basis should health be discounted? *Journal of Health Economics* 12, 39–53.

Oregon Health Services Commission. (1991). *Prioritization of Health Services: A Report to the Governor and Legislature*. Portland: Author.

Orentlicher, D. (1994). Rationing and the Americans with Disabilities Act. *Journal of the American Medical Association* 271, 308–314.

Pauker, S.G. & B.J. McNeil. (1981). Impact of patient preferences on the selection of therapy. *Journal of Chronic Diseases* 34, 77–86.

Pauly, M.V. (1968). The economics of moral hazard. *American Economic Review* 58, 231–237.

Pearson, T.A. (1998). Lipid-lowering therapy in low-risk patients. *Journal of the American Medical Association* 279, 1659–1660.

Pellegrino, E.D. (1979). Toward a reconstruction of medical morality: The primacy of the act of profession and the fact of illness. *Journal of Medicine and Philosophy* 4, 32.

Phelps, C.E. (1992). *Health Economics*. New York: HarperCollins.

Prades, J.-L.P. (1997). Is the person trade-off a valid method for allocating health care resources? *Health Economics* 6, 71–81.

Rawles, J. (1971). *A Theory of Justice*. Cambridge: Harvard University Press.

Rawles, J. (1989). Castigating QALYs. *Journal of Medical Ethics* 15, 143–147.

Read, J.L., R.J. Quinn, D.M. Berwick, et al. (1984). Preferences for health outcomes: Comparison of assessment methods. *Medical Decision Making* 4, 315–329.

Read, L., T.M. Pass, & A.L. Komaroff. (1982). Diagnosis and treatment of dyspepsia: A cost-effectiveness analysis. *Medical Decision Making* 2, 415–438.

Redelmeier, D.A. & D.N. Heller. (1993). Time preference in medical decision making and cost-effectiveness analysis. *Medical Decision Making* 13, 212–217.

Redelmeier, D.A, P. Rozin, & D. Kahneman. (1993). Understanding patients' decisions: Cognitive and emotional perspectives. *Journal of the American Medical Association* 270, 72–76.

Reinhardt, U.E. (1996). Economics. *Journal of the American Medical Association* 275, 1802–1803.

Reinhardt, U.E. (1997). Wanted: A clearly articulated social ethic for American health care. *Journal of the American Medical Association* 278, 1446–1446.

Reitemeier, P.J. & H. Brody. (1988). Treatment refusal for economic reasons. In J.F. Monagle & D.C. Thomasma (Eds.), *Medical Ethics: A Guide for Health Care Professionals*. Rockville, MD: Aspen Press.

Relman, A.S. (1990a). Is rationing inevitable? *New England Journal of Medicine* 322, 1809–1810.

Relman, A.S. (1990b). The trouble with rationing. *New England Journal of Medicine* 323, 911–913.

Richardson, J. (1994). Cost utility analysis: What should be measured? *Social Science and Medicine* 39, 7–21.

Robinson, J.C., L.B. Gardner, & H.S. Luft. (1993). Health plan switching in anticipation of increased medical care utilization. *Medical Care* 31, 43–51.

Russell, L.B., M.R. Gold, J.E. Siegel, & N. Daniels. (1996). The role of cost-effectiveness analysis in health and medicine. *Journal of the American Medical Association* 276, 1172–1177.

Sarin, R.K. (1985). Measuring equity in public risk. *Operations Research* 33, 210–217.

Schectman, J.M., E.G. Elinsky, & L.G. Pawlson. (1991). Effect of education and feedback on thyroid function testing strategies of primary care clinicians. *Archives of Internal Medicine* 151, 2163–2166.

Schelling, T.C. (1984). *Choice and Consequence: Perspectives of an Errant Economist*. Harvard University Press, Cambridge.

Schneiderman, L.J., N.S. Jecker, & A.R. Jonsen. (1990). Medical futility: Its meaning and ethical implications. *Annals of Internal Medicine* 112, 949–954.

Singer, M.G. (1971). *Generalization in Ethics: An Essay in the Logic of Ethics, with the Rudiments of a System of Moral Philosophy*. New York: Atheneum.

Singer, P.A., E.S. Tasch, C. Stocking, et al. (1991). Sex or survival: Trade-offs between quality and quantity of life. *Journal of Clinical Oncology* 9, 328–334.

Sloan, F.A., G.S. Gordon, & D.L. Cocks. (1993). Hospital drug formularies and use of hospital services. *Medical Care* 31, 851–867.

Society of Critical Care Medicine Ethics Committee. (1994). Attitudes of critical care medicine professionals concerning distribution of intensive care resources. *Critical Care Medicine* 22, 358–362.

Spiegel, J.S., M.F. Shapiro, B. Berman, & S. Greenfield. (1989). Changing physician test ordering in a university hospital: An intervention of physician participation, explicit criteria, and feedback. *Archives of Internal Medicine* 149, 549–553.

Steinberg, E.P., R.D. Moore, N.R. Powe, et al. (1992). Safety and cost effectiveness of high-osmolality as compared with low-osmolality contrast material in patients undergoing cardiac angiography. *New England Journal of Medicine* 326, 425–430.

Sullivan, L.W. (1992). Letter to Gov. Barbara Roberts. Washington, DC: U.S. Department of Health and Human Services.

Sulmasy, D.P. (1992). Physicians, cost control, and ethics. *Annals of Internal Medicine* 116, 920–926.

Tengs, T.O., M.E. Adams, J.S. Pliskin, et al. (1995). Five-hundred life-saving interventions and their cost-effectiveness. *Risk Analysis* 15, 369–390.

Torrance, G.W. (1986). Measurement of health state utilities for economic appraisal: A review. *Journal of Health Economics* 5, 1–30.

Torrance, G.W. (1976). Social preferences for health states: An empirical evaluation of three measurement techniques. *Socioeconomics Planning Science* 10, 129–136.

Truog, R.D, A.S. Brett, & J. Frader. (1992). The problem with futility. *New England Journal of Medicine* 326, 1560–1564.

Ubel, P.A. (1996). Informed consent: From bodily invasion to the seemingly mundane. *Archives of Internal Medicine* 156, 1262–1263.

Ubel, P.A., & R.M. Arnold. (1995). The unbearable rightness of bedside rationing: Physician duties in a climate of cost containment. *Archives of Internal Medicine* 155, 1837–1842.

Ubel, P.A., R.M. Arnold, & A.L. Caplan. (1993). Rationing failure: The ethical lessons of the retransplantation of scarce, vital organs. *Journal of the American Medical Association* 270, 2469–2474.

Ubel, P.A., J. Baron, & D.A. Asch. (1999). Social acceptability, personal responsibility, and prognosis in public judgments about transplant allocation. *Bioethics* 13, 57–68.

Ubel, P.A. & A.L. Caplan. (1998). Geographic favoritism in liver transplantation: Unfortunate or unfair? *New England Journal of Medicine* 339, 1322–1325.

Ubel, P.A., M.L. DeKay, J. Baron, & D.A. Asch. (1996a). Cost-effectiveness analysis in a setting of budget constraints: Is it equitable? *New England Journal of Medicine* 334, 1174–1177.

Ubel, P.A., M.L. DeKay, J. Baron, & D.A. Asch. (1996b). Public preferences for efficiency and racial equity in kidney transplant allocation decisions. *Transplantation Proceedings* 28, 2975–2980.

Ubel, P.A. & S.D. Goold. (1997). Recognizing bedside rationing: Clear cases and tough calls. *Annals of Internal Medicine* 126, 74–80.

Ubel, P.A. & G. Loewenstein. (1995). The efficacy and equity of retransplantation: An experimental survey of public attitudes. *Health Policy* 34, 145–151.

Ubel, P.A. & G. Loewenstein. (1996a). Distributing scarce livers: The moral reasoning of the general public. *Social Science and Medicine* 42, 1049–1055.

Ubel, P.A. & G. Loewenstein. (1996b). Public perceptions of the importance of prognosis in allocating transplantable livers to children. *Medical Decision Making* 16, 234–241.

Ubel, P.A. & G. Loewenstein. (1997). The role of decision analysis in informed consent: Choosing between intuition and systematicity. *Social Science and Medicine* 44, 647–656.

Ubel, P.A., G. Loewenstein, D. Scanlon, & M. Kamlet. (1998a). Value measurement in cost-utility analysis: Explaining the discrepancy between analog scale and person trade-off elicitations. *Health Policy* 43, 33–44.

Ubel, P.A., D. Scanlon, G. Loewenstein, & M. Kamlet. (1996c). Individual utilities are inconsistent with rationing choices: A partial explanation of why Oregon's cost-effectiveness list failed. *Medical Decision Making* 16, 108–119.

Ubel, P.A., M. Spranca, M. DeKay, et al. (1998b). Public preferences for prevention versus cure: What if an ounce of prevention is worth only an ounce of cure? *Medical Decision Making* 18, 141–148.

U.S. Preventive Services Task Force. (1996). *Guide to Clinical Preventive Services* (2nd ed.). Baltimore: Williams & Wilkins.

Veatch, R.M. (1981). *A Theory of Medical Ethics.* New York: Basic Books.

Viberti, G., C.E. Mogensen, L.C. Groop, & J.F. Pauls. (1994). Effect of captopril on progression to clinical proteinuria in patients with insulin-dependent diabetes mellitus and microalbuminuria. *Journal of the American Medical Association* 271, 275–279.

Weeks, J.C., M. Tierney, & M. Weinstein. (1991). Cost effectiveness of prophylactic intravenous immune globulin in chronic lymphocytic leukemia. *New England Journal of Medicine* 325, 81–86.

Weingarten, S.R., M.S. Riedinger, L. Conner, et al. (1994). Practice guidelines and reminders to reduce duration of hospital stay for patients with chest pain: An interventional trial. *Annals of Internal Medicine* 120, 257–263.

Weinstein, M.C. (1986). Challenges for cost-effectiveness research. *Medical Decision Making* 6, 194–198.

Welch, H.G. & E.B. Larson. (1988). Dealing with limited resources: The Oregon decision to curtail funding for organ transplantation. *New England Journal of Medicine* 319, 171–173.

Wennberg, J. & A. Gittelsohn. (1982). Variations in medical care among small areas. *Scientific American* 246, 120.

Wennberg, J.E., A.G. Mulley Jr., D. Hanley, et al. (1988). An assessment of prostatectomy for benign urinary tract obstruction: Geographic variations and the evaluation of medical care outcomes. *Journal of the American Medical Association* 259, 3027–3030.

Whittle, J., J. Conigliaro, C.B. Good, & R. Lofgren. (1993). Racial differences in the use of invasive cardiovascular procedures in the Department of Veterans Affairs medical system. *New England Journal of Medicine* 329, 621–627.

Williams, A. (1988). Ethics and efficiency in the provision of health care. In J. Bell & S. Mendus (Eds.), *Philosophy and Medical Welfare.* Cambridge: Cambridge University Press.

Williams, A. (1992). Cost-effectiveness analysis: Is it ethical? *Journal of Medical Ethics* 18, 7–11.

Winikoff, R.N., K.L. Coltin, M.M. Morgan, et al. (1984). Improving physician performance through peer comparison feedback. *Medical care* 22, 527–534.

Winslow, G.R. (1982). *Triage and Justice* Berkeley: University of California Press.

Wolf, A., J.F. Nasser, A.M. Wolf, & J.B. Scholring. (1996). The impact of informed consent on patient interest in prostate-specific antigen screening. *Archives of Internal Medicine* 156, 1333–1336.

Wolf, S.M. (1994). Health care reform and the future of physician ethics. *Hastings Center Report* 24, 28–41.

Yaari, M.E. & M. Bar-Hillel. (1984). On dividing justly. *Social Choice and Welfare* 1, 1–24.

Zweibel, N.R., C.K. Cassel, & T. Karrison. (1993). Public attitudes about the use of chronological age as a criterion for allocating health care resources. *Gerontologist* 33, 74–80.

Index

Note that figures are indicated by an italic *f* and tables are indicated by an italic *t* after the page number.